AF332946

DEEP VEIN THROMBOSIS

SYMPTOMS, DIAGNOSIS AND TREATMENTS

RECENT ADVANCES IN HEMATOLOGY RESEARCH

Additional books in this series can be found on Nova's website under the Series tab.

Additional e-books in this series can be found on Nova's website under the e-book tab.

RECENT ADVANCES IN HEMATOLOGY RESEARCH

DEEP VEIN THROMBOSIS

SYMPTOMS, DIAGNOSIS AND TREATMENTS

TAKASHI YAMAKI
EDITOR

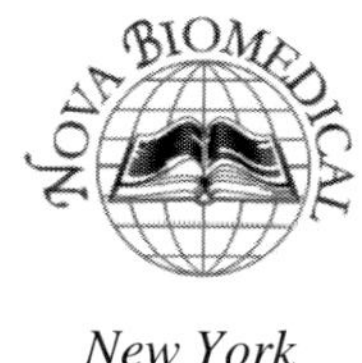

New York

For permission to use material from this book please contact us:
Telephone 631-231-7269; Fax 631-231-8175
Web Site: http://www.novapublishers.com

NOTICE TO THE READER

Library of Congress Cataloging-in-Publication Data

ISBN: 978-1-62257-519-0
Library of Congress Control Number: 2012942455

Published by Nova Science Publishers, Inc. † New York

Contents

Preface

Deep venous thrombosis (DVT) is the third most common cardiovascular disease. Two-thirds of patients with DVT are first episodes, and the remainders are recurrences. Pulmonary embolism is the most common complication of DVT. And now, DVT and pulmonary are considered two spectra of the same disease, namely venous thromboembolism (VTE). This book provides a comprehensive review of current diagnosis and treatment of DVT. This book includes chapters on clinical approaches in DVT, VTE and cancer, prevention of DVT in neurological surgery, combination of pretest clinical probability score and different D-dimer cutoff value for exclusion of VTE, ambulatory therapy for DVT, management of DVT with oral anticoagulant, surgical intervention for acute DVT, and recent multicenter survey of DVT from Japan. In this book, the mechanisms of VTE, diagnostic strategy of DVT, various treatment options for DVT, and prevention of VTE are discussed.

Chapter 1 - Deep venous thrombosis (DVT) is part of disease called venous thromboembolism (VTE) and is a life threatening condition that can lead to death. The annual incidence is 67 per 100,000 among general population. The primary mechanism is the Virchow triad, which are venous stasis, vessel wall injury, and hypercoagulable state. A balance between thrombogenesis and the body's protective mechanisms (inhibitors of coagulation and the fibrinolytic system) has the important role of venous thrombosis incidence. There are several factors that might contribute to this event, such as genetic factors, and acquired factors (long-haul air travel, cigarette smoking, pregnancy, obesity, oral contraceptive, post-menopausal hormone replacement, surgery, trauma, and others medical conditions like antiphospholipid antibody syndrome, cancer, hypertension, and chronic pulmonary obstructive disease). The clinical evaluation is very challenging since the symptoms and signs are non-specific. Patients usually have a cramp in the lower calf that persists for several days. Physical findings can shows mild palpation discomfort in the lower calf. In massive DVT, patient presents severe thigh swelling and marked tenderness when palpating the inguinal area and common femoral vein. The diagnosis can be established via clinical prediction rules, D-dimer (a degradation product of a cross-linked fibrin blood clot) testing, and imaging examination like compression ultrasonography with Doppler. It has been well established that a clinical prediction rule that takes into account signs, symptoms and risk factors can be applied to categorize patients as having low, moderate or high probability of DVT. The differential diagnoses for DVT are ruptured Baker's cyst, cellulitis, and post-phlebitic syndrome/venous insufficiency. The main goal of DVT management is to prevent the extension of thrombus and pulmonary embolism in the short-term and to prevent recurrent events in the long-term. The standard therapy for DVT is heparin (unfractionated heparin/UFH or low molecular weight heparin/LMWH). The advantage of UFH is that it has a short half-life. Its anticoagulant effect abates after several hours. The disadvantage of UFH is that achieving aPTT target can be difficult and may require repeated blodd sampling and heparin dose adjustment every 4-6 hours. The route of administration and efficacy of LMWH make this the preferred anticoagulant. Based on a meta-analysis comparing the effectiveness of LMWH at a fixed dose with UFH at an adjusted dose, significantly fewer deaths, major hemorrhages and recurrent venous thromboembolisms occurred with the LMWH.

Chapter 2 – A venous thromboembolism is a common complication in patients with cancer, and it is associated with high morbidity, mortality, medical care and costs. Classical clinical symptoms of DVT are: pain, unilateral edema and heaviness in the distal extremity to the site of the venous thrombosis or edema in the face, neck or supraclavicular space. These signs and symptoms are not present in all cases so the diagnosis of DVT and PE made on clinical ground alone is notoriously unreliable. A clinical suspicion for VTE requires sensitive imaging studies such as a color duplex ultrasonography, spiral chest CT and ventilation-perfusion scan; in some cases, CT or MR venography could be useful. VTE risk factors in cancer patients are related to the type and stage of tumors, to the characteristics of patients (age, familial or acquired hypercoagulability, medical comorbidities, performance status) and to the treatment (surgery, chemotherapy, endocrine therapy, insertion of central venous catheter). Modifiable risk factors are obesity, smoking history and exercise. Currently available drugs for preventing and treatingVTE are vitamin K antagonists (VKA), unfractioned heparin (UFH) and low molecular weight heparins (LMWHs). New antithrombotic agents, such as oral IIa and Xa inhibitors, could be useful, but further studies are needed.

Chapter 3 – *Background*: The mean incidence of deep vein thrombosis (DVT) in neurosurgical reports is variable and surprisingly approaches 25%, whereas the incidence of pulmonary embolism (PE) is thought to be between 1.5% and 3%, with a mortality rate between 9% and 50%. Although DVT is probably the single most important, preventable cause of morbidity and mortality in this domain, its pharmacologic prevention is still a controversial matter due to the concern associated with the possible increased risk of postoperative haemorrhaging. Prophylactic options against DVT/PE include elastic stockings, intermittent pneumatic compression devices, low-dose unfractionated heparin (UFH), and low molecular-weight heparin (LMWH). The aim of this chapter is to describe the prophylactic protocols for DVT currently in use in neurological surgery and share our experience on this topic.

Analysis of the prophylactic protocols in neurological surgery: Systematic reviews of the English literature concerning DVT prophylactic protocols in neurosurgery have been conducted by a PubMed search (back to 1986). at the latter aimed to analyze the risks and benefits associated with different prophylactic regimens: abstracts of all identified articles were reviewed, and detailed information from eligible articles was extracted.

Description of our own protocol: Herein, we describe the DVT prophylactic protocol currently in use at the Neurosurgical Department in Trieste (Italy) and report the related results obtained on more than 3,818 consecutive patients that have undergone neurosurgical cranial or spinal procedures at our institution since January 2004. All patients were screened with preoperative blood coagulation tests.According to the presence of risk factors in the anamnesis, the type of surgical procedure (minor or major cranial or spinal procedures) and expectations associated with their postoperative course (prolonged immobilization), the patients were then stratified into three classes of risk: low-, moderate- or high-risk subgroups. The protocol is associated with both pharmacological and mechanical prophylactic measures: administering LMWH (2,000 UI to 4,000 UI per day), elasting stockings and mechanical pneumatic sequential compression leg devices. The end points of this protocol are to keep the incidence of DVT, PE and postoperative haemorrhaging as low as possible. Over the years, they were assessed as follows: in the case of neurological deterioration, significant bleeding in the surgical site was promptly ruled out by a head or spinal CT scan, as well in the case of a clinical suspicion for DVT or PE, a duplex ultrasonography and a chest x-ray plus a perfusion CT scan were respectively performed.

Results: Although literature confirms that intermittent pneumatic compression devices provide an adequate reduction of DVT/PE in some cranial and combined cranial/spinal series, UFH or LMWH have proved to further reduce the incidence of PE, and partially reduce the incidence of DVT. Nevertheless, UFH-based prophylaxis showed a higher incidence of postoperative haemorrhaging (2% - 4% in cranial series, and 1% in spinal ones), whereas LMWH protocols present less bleeding drawbacks. Our prophylactic protocol was well tolerated in all patients; particularly the stratification of risk and subdivision into risk groups gave us the opportunity to avoid concerns regarding overtreatment. Clinical evidence of DVT occurred in 0.4% of our cohort; one patient died of fatal PE 2 months after surgery. Less than 1% of our patients presented significant postoperative haemorrhaging, mostly after major cranial surgery.

Conclusion: The results reported in literature confirm the need for a DVT prophylactic protocol in neurosurgical patients: a combined mechanical/pharmacological regimen seems to be the most appropriate and effective, but a prospective randomized trial to assess the best dosage, molecule and timing of LMWH administration is still lacking. On the other hand, even if our database only allows for an observational analysis, the results obtained in such a large group of neurosurgical patients are encouraging, since they show the efficacy in terms of DVT and PE prevention, without significant incidence of postoperative complications such as surgical-site haemorrhaging. Certainly, this data gives enough evidence to support the DVT prophylactic protocol applied throughout the last 6 years at our institution.

Chapter 4 – Prompt diagnosis of venous deep vein thromboembolism (VTE) is mandatory, but only 25% of suspected cases are confirmed by objective testing. In this background, the D-dimer testing with high negative predictive value represents an excellent triage test in patients with suspected VTE. In general, enzyme-liked immunosorbent assay (ELISA) offers the best of current D-dimer assay for sensitivity. Latex quantitative assay and whole-blood assay might also represent valid alternative for exclusion of VTE. Recently, a combination of pretest clinical probability (PTP) score and D-dimer testing has been considered validated as a diagnostic strategy for pulmonary embolism or deep vein thrombosis (DVT). This strategy is specifically validated for patients who have low PTP. Even the combination of low PTP and a normal D-dimer concentration can be considered a safe strategy to withhold anticoagulation in patients with suspected VTE.

D-dimer cutoff value also affects the discriminating power. The sensitivity could be improved by lowering the cutoff value, but the subsequent decrease in specificity would lead to a large number of false-positive results. On the contrary, D-dimer assays with very high specificity provide fewer false-positive results, but they are less sensitive for VTE and cannot be used to exclude the disease in all patients. In this background, the authors analyzed if varying the D-dimer cutoff according to PTP would exclude VTE in more patients than using the single D-dimer cutoff point. Using latex agglutination assay, the authors found that D-dimer cutoff points of 2.6, 1.1 and 1.1µg/mL were selected for the low, moderate and high PTP groups among 886 patients with suspected DVT. In the low PTP group, specificity increased from 48.9% to 78.2% (P <0.0001) with use of the different D-dimer cutoff value. In the moderate and high risk PTP groups, however, the different D-dimer levels did not achieve substantial improvement. Regardless, overall venous duplex scanning could have been reduced by 43.0% using different D-dimer cutoff points. Even in patients with proven PE, a combination of a specific D-dimer level and PTP score is most effective in the low PTP patients in excluding DVT.

In summary, a combination of PTP score and different D-dimer cutoff provides an effective means in terms of avoiding a large number of unnecessary venous duplex scanning in suspected symptomatic DVT in the low PTP for DVT.

Chapter 5 – Various options are available for the treatment of deep vein thrombosis (DVT) while the natural course of the disease without intervention results in 30% pulmonary embolus and 10% mortality.

Despite the evident consensus on the high efficacy of anticoagulant and thrombolytic treatments in the prevention of pulmonary embolus in the scientific era, these treatment options are known to be less effective in the prevention of post-thrombotic syndrome (PTS) which is another potential complication. In this respect, thrombolytic treatment has become the main therapeutic option recommended for ilio-femoral DVT which has been considered associated with higher PTS possibility. However, since the past clinical trials on ambulatory conservative anticoagulant treatment were based on the old literature during the former decade, comparison of this treatment with the recent thrombolytic treatment approach seems to be neither reasonable nor appropriate. Furthermore, there are no randomized clinical trials concerning the direct comparison of thrombolytic and anticoagulant treatments as of yet. Attractive trial results will be published soon but they may also not be able to answer all of the questions.

In this regard, the authors performed a clinical multi-center study based on an 18-month follow-up of 250 patients in order to evaluate the clinical outcome of neglected ambulatory conservative treatment in detail. According to the results of this study, conservative treatment was determined to be an effective and successful treatment alternative, associated with high total re-canalization ratios reaching 80%, especially in ilio-femoral DVT. When considered in terms of PTS, conservative treatment was also associated with high patient satisfaction with respect to complaints of the patients. For these reasons, the authors declare conventional conservative treatment to be the most ideal alternative in consensus meeting having level of evidence 1A with comparable and even preferable results in terms of better cost-effectiveness to thrombolytic treatment.

Chapter 6 – Oral vitamin K antagonist therapy is useful for prevention and treatment of thromboembolic disease. The fear of medication errors and medication related adverse events limit the appropriate use of oral vitamin k antagonist therapy. The beneficial effectiveness of oral vitamin K antagonist therapy depends on the adequate dose and its long term management. Acenocoumarol and warfarin are the commonly used vitamin K antagonists (VKAs) in our practice. Long term management (6 months) of the DVT patients with vitamin K antagonists has increased in recent years with improvement in the diagnostic methods of DVT detection and increasing age of the population. The pharmacokinetic and pharmacodynamic properties of the vitamin K antagonists along with the narrow therapeutic range make the management of oral anticoagulation for thromboembolic complications complex. Patients receiving oral anticoagulants are likely to attend emergency department due to bleeding from the medication errors. So, this is a serious concern in many countries and one would like to avoid the medication errors by maintaining the high quality of anticoagulation in DVT patients. During the initiation of oral anticoagulation therapy injection of heparin and oral anticoagulants are overlapped till the therapeutic INR values are achieved with the vitamin K antagonists. This overlap is maintained till two consecutive INR values are above 2.0. The authors generally start oral anticoagulation with 5mgs of tablet warfarin or 4mgs of tablet Acitrom as the higher doses are known to precipitate early hemorrhages. In the elderly people, undernourished, heart failure, liver disease and postoperative patients the anticoagulation is initiated with smaller doses (<5 mgs) due to the fear of bleeding. CYP2C9 is the principal enzyme to metabolize the oral anticoagulants and polymorphisms of the gene coding CYP2C9 can result in abnormalities. Recent studies are showing the advantages of pharmacogenetic based dosing to overcome these abnormalities, but it is not yet widely accepted or recommended. The warfarin inhibits the vitamin K oxide reductase complex (VKORC) and mutation of the genes coding this enzyme complex (VKORC1) can increase the sensitivity or resistance to warfarin inhibition. The adequate therapeutic dose to maintain INR shows variability due to these mutations. The therapeutic anticoagulation (INR>2) should be maintained to get maximum benefit. That means the time in therapeutic range (TTR) correlates with the clinical outcomes of hemorrhage and thrombosis. Increased TTR has also been associated with decreased mortality. INR test is performed at regular intervals of 7-14 days depending on the stable dose response in a given patient. Management of non-therapeutic INR is difficult in patients with complex life styles and variable dietary habits. Non-compliance and concomitant medications makes this more difficult to manage and maintain the therapeutic INRs. The target therapeutic INRs can be achieved by adjusting the warfarin doses with up or down increments of 5-20% and frequent monitoring. When the INR is between 4-10 without bleeding it is better to stop the medication and monitor the INR daily and restart with the reduced weekly dose of INR after it has fallen to the therapeutic range. Abnormally elevated INRs with or without bleeding would need attention and careful follow up adjustment of doses. The authors are cautious in correcting the abnormally high INRs associated with bleeding with Vitamin K injections which can increase the vitamin K resistance to warfarin later. Correction dose requirements are dependent on age, race, BMI, concomitant medications, co-morbidities and gene mutations. Systematic reviews of the patients on warfarin have shown bleeding rates of 8.9% per patient year in first 3 months, only 2.5% after 3 months of initiation of anticoagulation therapy. When patients are actively bleeding while they are on oral vitamin K antagonists one would target rapid lowering of the INRs with infusion of fresh frozen plasma (FFP), Prothrombin concentrates or recombinant factor VIIa along with injection vitamin K to facilitate the endogenous coagulation factor production. Quality patient education is necessary to achieve the safe and effective oral anticoagulation with Vitamin K antagonists under the supervision of the treating teams. It is indeed a challenge for the teams providing the oral anticoagulation therapies to prevent the recurrent thrombosis and thromboembolism in deep vein thrombosis in patients in many countries through quality education of patients to achieve the maximum time in therapeutic range.

Chapter 7 – The ilio-femoral venous thrombosis has higher risks of fatal pulmonary embolism, severe pain and swelling, moreover developing ischemia of the affected leg. In addition, the disabling post-thrombotic syndrome (PTS) which causes the pain, swelling, pigmentation or ulceration of legs is often found as late complications. The anticoagulant therapy is a widely accepted treatment for acute deep vein thrombosis to prevent pulmonary embolism and recurrent deep vein thrombosis with strong evidence. However, the results of anticoagulants are not always satisfied from the points of eliminating patient's complaints quickly and further prevention of PTS. Several reports show that the early removal of venous thrombus plays an important role of maintaining venous valvular competence and preventing PTS. So catheter-directed thrombolysis (CDT) and surgical thrombectomy, which can be expected, and early removal of venous thrombus are considered aggressive treatments of ilio-femoral venous thrombosis to relieve symptom quickly and prevent post-thrombotic syndrome more than anticoagulant therapy alone. Since the excellent thrombolytic result of CDT was reported with less invasive, venous thrombectomy is becoming an alternative method of CDT. Currently, the surgical thrombectomy tends to be indicated for mobilized patients who have acute ilio-femoral thrombus with the contraindication or failure of thrombolysis.

Thrombectomy for ilio-femoral venous thrombosis is approached from the common femoral vein using a Fogarty catheter and manual massage under general anesthesia with the protection of peri-operative pulmonary thromboembolism. The construction of temporary A-V fistula and additional endovenous procedures such as stenting for the stenotic iliac vein are recommended to maintain the patency of the ilio-femoral vein.

Previous reports show the early and late results of surgical thrombectomy with selected indications are fairly good. The surgical thrombectomy is still an option for the treatment of severe acute ilio-femoral vein thrombosis.

Chapter 8 – Several years have passed since the guidelines of venous thromboembolism (VTE) treatment and VTE prevention were published. The treatment of deep vein thrombosis (DVT) is changing greatly. This study was performed to investigate the risk factors, diagnostic methods, distribution, and treatment of DVT and to investigate VTE prevention in Japan.

A questionnaire survey was mailed to the members of the Japanese Society of Phlebology. The contents of the survey dealt with the treatment of new DVT cases in the year 2009 and the prevention of VTE. The results were examined and compared to the result of our former survey.

1162 patients were reported from 70 institutions. The sex ratio (men to women) was 1 to 2 and the age ranged from 15 to 102 (average 69). Surgery was the most important risk factor for DVT (38.2%). As for the onset time, the acute onset (within 13 days) occurred in 486 patients (41.8%) and the subacute (14-29 days) in 70 (6.0%). Subsequent pulmonary thromboembolism was diagnosed in 174 patients (15.0%). For diagnosis, an ultrasound method was mainly used (87.7%), whereas phlebography was used for only 33 patients (2.8%). DVT was found in left lower limb in 531 patients (48.6%), in right lower limb in 360 patients (33.0%) and in bilateral limbs in 201 patients (18.4%). DVT locations were proximal type (52.2%) and distal type (47.8%), which included 119 patients with bilateral distal type. In the distal type, soleal vein thrombosis was most frequent (84.3%) and then peroneal vein thrombosis (19.9%). Patients were mainly treated medicinally (80.8%). Medication included unfractionated heparin (57.0%) and Urokinase (11.1%). Catheter-directed thrombectomy was performed in 22 cases (2.4%) and surgical thrombectomy was done only in 14 (1.6%). Vena cava filter was inserted for 155 patients (17.2%): retrievable type (66.5%), permanent type (21.3%) and temporary type (9.7%). Prophylactic methods were used at 60 institutions (85.7%). The precautions were elastic stockings (91.4%), early ambulation (84.3%), pneumatic compression (81.4%) and anticoagulant drugs (52.9%).

The number of DVT patients has increased and the frequency of the distal type especially increased. Anticoagulant therapy is most common medical treatment. The total frequency of vena cava filter was similar to our previous survey; however, the use ratio of retrievable type increased comparatively. Prophylactic methods for VTE were used in most institutions, however, the rate of anticoagulation administration was not high and is considered to be insufficient in Japan.

In: Deep Vein Thrombosis
Editor: Takashi Yamaki

ISBN: 978-1-62257-519-0
© 2013 Nova Science Publishers, Inc.

Chapter 1

Clinical Approach in Deep Vein Thrombosis

C. Rinaldi A. Lesmana and Aru W. Sudoyo[*]
Department of Internal Medicine, Cipto Mangunkusumo Hospital,
Medical Faculty, University of Indonesia, Jakarta, Indonesia

Abstract

Deep venous thrombosis (DVT) is part of disease called venous
thromboembolism (VTE) and is a life threatening condition that can lead
to death. The annual incidence is 67 per 100,000 among general
population. The primary mechanism is the Virchow triad, which are
venous stasis, vessel wall injury, and hypercoagulable state. A balance
between thrombogenesis and the body's protective mechanisms
(inhibitors of coagulation and the fibrinolytic system) has the important
role of venous thrombosis incidence. There are several factors that might
contribute to this event, such as genetic factors, and acquired factors
(long-haul air travel, cigarette smoking, pregnancy, obesity, oral
contraceptive, post-menopausal hormone replacement, surgery, trauma,
and others medical conditions like antiphospholipid antibody syndrome,
cancer, hypertension, and chronic pulmonary obstructive disease). The

---

[*] Correspondence to: C. Rinaldi A. Lesmana M.D. Department of Internal Medicine, Cipto
Mangunkusumo Hospital Medical Faculty, University of Indonesia, Diponegoro St. No.71,
Kenari Village, Senen, Central Jakarta City, 10430 Indonesia. Tel: +62-21-391-8301. E-
mail: medicaldr2001id@yahoo.com.

clinical evaluation is very challenging since the symptoms and signs are non-specific. Patients usually have a cramp in the lower calf that persists for several days. Physical findings can shows mild palpation discomfort in the lower calf. In massive DVT, patient presents severe thigh swelling and marked tenderness when palpating the inguinal area and common femoral vein. The diagnosis can be established via clinical prediction rules, D-dimer (a degradation product of a cross-linked fibrin blood clot) testing, and imaging examination like compression ultrasonography with Doppler. It has been well established that a clinical prediction rule that takes into account signs, symptoms and risk factors can be applied to categorize patients as having low, moderate or high probability of DVT. The differential diagnoses for DVT are ruptured Baker's cyst, cellulitis, and post-phlebitic syndrome/venous insufficiency. The main goal of DVT management is to prevent the extension of thrombus and pulmonary embolism in the short-term and to prevent recurrent events in the long-term. The standard therapy for DVT is heparin (unfractionated heparin/UFH or low molecular weight heparin/LMWH). The advantage of UFH is that it has a short half-life. Its anticoagulant effect abates after several hours. The disadvantage of UFH is that achieving aPTT target can be difficult and may require repeated blodd sampling and heparin dose adjustment every 4-6 hours. The route of administration and efficacy of LMWH make this the preferred anticoagulant. Based on a meta-analysis comparing the effectiveness of LMWH at a fixed dose with UFH at an adjusted dose, significantly fewer deaths, major hemorrhages and recurrent venous thromboembolisms occurred with the LMWH.

Introduction

Deep Vein Thrombosis (DVT) is a part of venous thromboembolism (VTE) and it is a serious clinical condition with life-threatening complications. It can be located either at the upper extremity (UEDVT) or lower extremities (proximal or distal). [1, 2] Even though DVT has been known very well for many years in clinical practice, it is still challenging to diagnose and perform the right management, especially where management in special conditions is needed.

Previous studies had reported that DVT incidence was higher than pulmonary embolism (PE) among all VTE incidences. The mortality rates increase as the PE developed during DVT incidence. Ethnicity has become a major risk factor for DVT development, which is highly found in Caucasians and African Americans. There are other several conditions (inherited/acquired) that can contribute to DVT development, such as antithrombin, protein C, protein S deficiency, Factor V Leiden mutation, G20210A prothrombin-gene mutation, dysfibrinogenemia, major surgery, antiphospholipid antibodies, cancer, age, pregnancy, hormonal therapy, obesity, and hyperhomocysteinemia.

Recent studies have shown that DVT could also occur in patients with advanced liver disease (hepatic cirrhosis). [1, 3, 4] Virchow's triad (vessel wall damage, venous stasis, hypercoagulability) is a well-known pathogenesis in DVT, but the venous stasis mechanism has not been cleared yet for many years until the role of VWF and platelet adhesions were showed in a recent study. In advanced liver disease, hypoalbuminemia, and the decrease of level protein C and S are thought has a role in DVT incidence. [1, 3, 4]

Sign and Symptoms

Patients with UEDVT are sometimes asymptomatic. Otherwise, patients can complain of vague shoulder or neck discomfort and arm edema. Besides arm and facial edema, the patients can suffer from head fullness, blurred vision, vertigo, or dyspnea whenever the thrombosis causes superior vena cava obstruction. Patients with thoracic outlet obstruction may have pain that radiates into the fourth and fifth digits via the medial arm and forearm, attributable to injury of the brachial plexus.

The signs can manifest as supraclavicular fullness, arm or hand edema, extremity cyanosis, dilated cutaneous vein, jugular venous distension, or unable to access central venous catheter (CVC). Brachial plexus tenderness, hand or arm atrophy, and positive Adson or Wright maneuver could be found when thoracic outlet syndrome occurred. [2, 5]

Lower extremity pain, tenderness, and swelling could be found in patients with lower extremity DVT. There are some other conditions that can mimic DVT at lower extremity.

Homans' sign (pain associated with forced dorsiflexion of the ankle) is often used as a sign to diagnose DVT. The patient's knee should be in the flexed position when evaluate the Homan's sign. There are several controversies in using Homan's sign since it can also be found in patients without DVT. Based on previous studies, the accuracy of using Homan's sign was found in only 8-56%. [2]

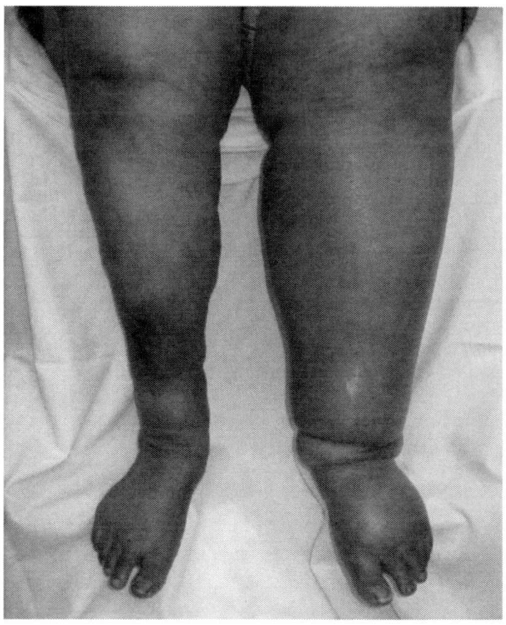

Figure 1. Example picture of patient with DVT.

Diagnosis

There are several methods that can be used to diagnose DVT, such as clinical diagnosis, Wells rule (Table 3), D-dimer test, Plethysmography, Doppler ultrasonography, helical CT, and venography. [6-10]

Wells rule is the most clinical prediction rule that has been used for many years to diagnose DVT. However, there are controversies using this rule with or without D-dimer combination. In one large cross-sectional study in primary care settings, it was shown that the prevalence of DVT using Wells rule with D-dimer combination in low risk population was higher compared to original study, even though the sensitivity increased. Another prospective study in primary care settings also found moderate to low sensitivity and poor specificity in using Wells rule alone to diagnose DVT. A review study found that combining the clinical prediction rules with D-dimer has a very high negative predictive value. [7, 8, 10] Plasma D-dimers are produced by fibrin when it is degraded by plasmin. This test alone is insufficient to make a diagnosis of DVT, especially whenever there are other conditions that also can influenced the level, such as pregnancy, malignancy, and after operations. One study found that a combination using a validated clinical prediction rule and a negative second-generation latex agglutination D-dimer assay effectively rule out the incidence of DVT. Based on assay type, D-dimer using ELISA has 95% sensitivity and 96% sensitivity for quantitative rapid ELISA to diagnose DVT. [7, 8, 10] There are three kinds of plethysmography; digital, computerized, and impedance. Digital pletysmography is assisted by a microprocessor. A digital measurement probe is placed on the skin, 10 cm above the medial malleolus of the affected leg. Then the patient dorsiflexes the foot 10 times according to a standard protocol and then rests for 45 seconds. The venous refilling time is calculated and presented as a printed graph. Based on one study, it has 100% sensitivity and 47% specificity. But it still needs a larger study to confirm these findings. The computerized strain gauge plethysmography measures the changes in calf dimensions while venous outflow is occluded by inflation of a thigh cuff.

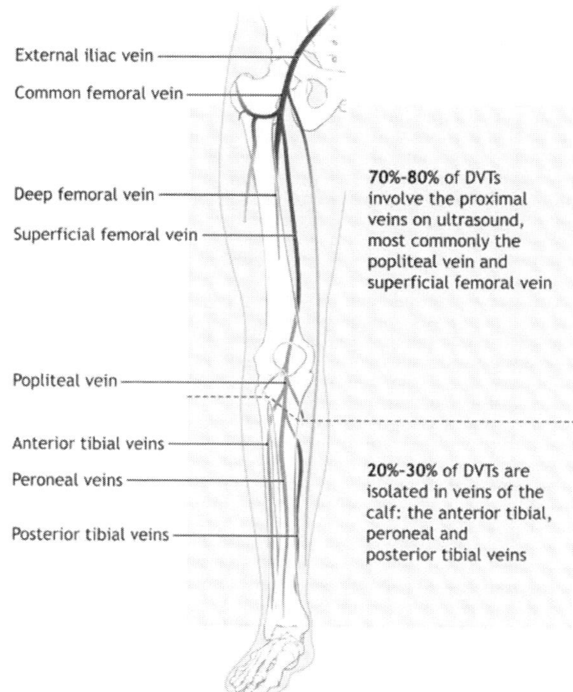

Derived from Scarvelis D et al. CMAJ 2006; 175:1087-92.

Figure 2. Diagram of leg veins.

Table 1. Risk Factors for Deep Venous Thrombosis[7]

Clinical Finding	Score[a]
Active cancer (within 6 months of diagnosis or palliative care)	1
Paralysis, paresis, or recent plaster immobilization of lower extremity	1
Recently bedridden >3 days or major surgery within 4 weeks of application Within 4 weeks of application of clinical decision rule	1
Localized tenderness along distribution of the deep venous system[b]	1
Entire lower extremity swelling	1
Calf swelling by >3 cm compared with asymptomatic lower extremity[c]	1
Pitting edema (greater in the symptomatic lower extremity)	1
Collateral superficial veins (nonvaricose)	1
Alternative diagnosis as likely as or greater than that of DVT[d]	-2

[a]Score interpretation: ≤ 0: probability of proximal lower extremity deep vein thrombosis (PDVT) of 3% (95% confidence interval (CI) 1.7-5.9%), 1 or 2: probability of PDVT of 17% (95% CI 12-23%), ≥ 3: probability of 75% (95% CI 63-84%).

[b]Tenderness along the deep venous system is assessed by deep palpation in the center of the posterior calf, the popliteal space, and along the area of the femoral vein in the anterior thigh and groin.

[c]Measured 10 cm below tibial tuberosity.

[d]Most common alternative diagnosis are cellulitis, calf strain, and post-operative swelling.

Calibration of the strain gauge and blood flow calculation are done by computer software. This test can be performed in 15 minutes and only minimal training is needed. One study has shown 99% sensitivity for proximal DVT and 66% sensitivity for distal DVT. The impedance pletysmography relies on the principle that the volume of blood in the leg affects the blood's ability to conduct an electrical current, which is inversely proportional to the impedance between two electrodes placed along the calf. When the blood accumulates in the leg below the cuff, impedance between the calf electrodes falls. The sudden release of the cuff results in a rapid increase in impedance due to the decrease of the blood volume. Since the sensitivity is low, some centers combine this measurement tool with the D-dimer test. [6]

Ultrasonography has been considered as the best non-invasive method to diagnose DVT, especially for proximal DVT as it has 97% sensitivity and specificity. However, only 75% sensitivity has been reported when using ultrasonography to diagnose calf vein thrombosis. There are three techniques in ultrasonography, which are compression ultrasound, duplex ultrasonography, and color flow duplex imaging. [9] Despite spiral computed tomography venography and magnetic resonance imaging that are still very costly, venography is still the gold standard to confirm the diagnosis of DVT. However, there are some risks such as allergic reaction or venous thrombosis as this is an invasive procedure. [9]

Treatment

Based on recent evidence, low molecular weight heparin (LMWH) is superior compared to unfractionated heparin (UFH) as an initial treatment for DVT. The LMWH is also safer and more cost-effective when compared to UFH when looking to the bleeding side effect and therapeutic level of achievement. Some studies also showed that using LMWH reduced the incidence of heparin-induced thrombocytopenia. Another treatment using pentasaccharide fondaparinux (newer agent) also has shown as effective as LMWH for DVT. This drug also can be used without body weight adjustment. International Consensus Statement Guideline 2006 also has recommended the use of fondaparinux as an initial treatment for DVT. [11, 12]

Table 2. Heparin Therapy for Deep Vein Thrombosis

Weight-Based Heparin Therapy with Adjustments Based on the APTT	
Initial dosage	Bolus of 80 U/Kg, then 18 U/Kg/h by infusion
APTT < 35 s (<1.2 x control)	Bolus 80 U/Kg, then 4 U/Kg/h by infusion
APTT = 35-45 s (1.2-1.5x control)	Bolus of 40 U/Kg, then 2 U/Kg/h by infusion
APTT = 46-70 s (1.5-2.3x control)	No Change
APTT = 71-90 s (2.0-3.0x control)	Decreased infusion rate by 2U/Kg/h
APTT >90 s (> 3.0x control)	Hold infusion by 1 h then decreased infusion rate by 3U/Kg/h

APTT: Activated Partial Thromboplastin Time.
Adapted from Raschke RA et al. Ann Intern Med 1993;119:875.

Vitamin K antagonist (VKA) is an oral anticoagulant which has been shown to be a very effective agent for long-term treatment depending on the risk for DVT recurrences. There are 5 risk categories, such as proximal DVT in transient risk factor (surgery or trauma) which is categorized as a low risk and only needs limited duration of therapy (3months), in the malignancy condition which is considered a longer duration of therapy (6 months), in the thrombophilic defect condition which has not been cleared enough for long duration of therapy, after second recurrence of DVT which is considered for more than 6 months duration of therapy, and idiopathic DVT which is considered a minimum of 6 months therapy. [13, 14]

Table 3. Low Molecular Weight Heparin (LMWH) Therapy[14]

LMWH	DOSE
Dalteparin	100 IU/kg SQ b.i.d. or 200 IU SQ q.d.
Enoxaparin	1.0 mg/kg b.i.d (studied in outpatients with/without PE) 1.5 mg/kg SQ q.d. (studied in inpatients with/without PE)
Tinzaparin	175 IU/kg SQ q.d. (acute treatment of DVT with/without PE)
PENTASACCHARIDE Fondaparinux	7.5 mq SQ q.d.
UFH SQ (non-dose adjusted)	333 IU/kg SQ initially, followed by 250 IU/kg SQ q12h
IV (weight-based nomogram)	80 U/kg initial bolus, followed by 18 U/kg/h maintenance

At least 5-day overlap with vitamin K antagonist until stable international normalized ratio (>2.0) achieved.

Special Populations

There are conditions which are considered as special populations, such as pregnancy and advanced liver disease. LMWH is the treatment of choice during pregnancy[12]. In advanced liver disease, there have not been a lot of studies yet to see the risk and benefit for long-term anticoagulants, especially after the first incidence of DVT.

References

[1]   Ramzi, D.W., Leeper, K.V. DVT and pulmonary embolism: Part I. Diagnosis. *Am. Fam. Physician.* 69, 2829-36 (2004).

[2]   Urbano, F.L. Homan's sign in the diagnosis of deep venous thrombosis. *Hospital. Physician.* 22-4 (2001).

[3]　Northup, P.G., McMahon, M.M., Ruhl, A.P., Aetschuler, S.E., Bednarz, A.V., Caldwell, S.H., Berg, C.L. Coagulopathy does not fully protect hospitalized cirrhosis patients from peripheral venous thromboembolism. *Am. J. Gastroenterol.* 101, 1524-8 (2006).

[4]　Lesmana, C.R.A., Inggriani, S., Cahyadinata, L., Lesmana, L.A. Deep vein thrombosis in patients with advanced liver cirrhosis: a rare condition? *Hepatol. Int.* 4, 433-8 (2010).

[5]　Joffe, H.V., Goldhaber, S.Z. Upper-extremity deep vein thrombosis. *Circulation.* 106, 1874-80 (2002).

[6]　Tovey, C., Wyatt, S. Diagnosis, investigation, and management of deep vein thrombosis. *BMJ.* 326, 1180-4 (2003).

[7]　Scarvelis, D., Wells, P.S. Diagnosis and treatment of deep vein thrombosis. *CMAJ.* 175, 1087-92 (2006).

[8]　Riddle, D.L., Wells, P.S. Diagnosis of lower extremity deep vein thrombosis in outpatients. *Phys. Ther.* 84, 729-35 (2004).

[9]　Fraser, J.D., Anderson, D.R. Deep venous thrombosis: Recent advances and optimal investigations with US. *Radiology.* 211, 9-24 (1999).

[10]　Qaseem, A., Snow, V., Barry, P., Hornbale, E.R., Rodnick, J.E., Tobolic, T., et al. Current diagnosis of venous thromboembolism in primary care: A clinical practice guideline from the American Academy of Family Physicians and the American College of Physicians. *Am. Fam. Med.* 5, 57-62 (2007).

[11]　Bates, S.M., Ginsberg, J.S. Treatment of deep vein thrombosis. *N. Engl. J. Med.* 351, 268-77 (2004).

[12]　Ramzi, D.W., Leeper, K.V. DVT and pulmonary embolism: Part II. Treatment and prevention. *Am. Fam. Physician.* 69, 2841-8 (2004).

[13]　Dentali, F., Douketis, J.D., Gianni, M., Lim, W., Crowther, M.A. Meta-analysis: Anticoagulant prophylaxis to prevent symptomatic venous thromboembolism in hospitalized medical patients. *Ann. Intern. Med.* 146, 278-88 (2007).

[14]　Garcia, D.A., Spyropoulos, A.C. Update in the treatment of venous thromboembolism. *Semin. Respir. Crit. Care. Med.* 29, 40-6 (2008).

Chapter 2

Thromboembolic Events and Cancer

Jennifer Foglietta, Stefania Gori, Lucia Stocchi and Lucio Crinò[*]
Medical Oncology Department,
S. Maria della Misericordia Hospital, Italy

Abstract

A venous thromboembolism is a common complication in patients
with cancer, and it is associated with high morbidity, mortality, medical
care and costs. Classical clinical symptoms of DVT are: pain, unilateral
edema and heaviness in the distal extremity to the site of the venous
thrombosis or edema in the face, neck or supraclavicular space. These
signs and symptoms are not present in all cases so the diagnosis of DVT
and PE made on clinical ground alone is notoriously unreliable. A clinical
suspicion for VTE requires sensitive imaging studies such as a color
duplex ultrasonography, spiral chest CT and ventilation-perfusion scan;
in some cases, CT or MR venography could be useful. VTE risk factors
in cancer patients are related to the type and stage of tumors, to the
characteristics of patients (age, familial or acquired hypercoagulability,

[*] Correspondence to: Jennifer Foglietta MD, Medical Oncology Department, S.Maria della
Misericordia Hospital, Via Dottori 1, 06126 Perugia, Italy. Tel: +39-075-578-4099. E-mail:
jennifer.foglietta@libero.it.

medical comorbidities, performance status) and to the treatment (surgery, chemotherapy, endocrine therapy, insertion of central venous catheter). Modifiable risk factors are obesity, smoking history and exercise. Currently available drugs for preventing and treatingVTE are vitamin K antagonists (VKA), unfractioned heparin (UFH) and low molecular weight heparins (LMWHs). New antithrombotic agents, such as oral IIa and Xa inhibitors, could be useful, but further studies are needed.

Epidemiology and Pathophysiology of Venous Thromboembolism

Venous thromboembolisms (VTEs) are a major source of morbidity and mortality for patients with cancer, with reported incidence rates ranging from 3.8% to 30.7% in comparison to an incidence of VTE of 2.5% in the general population. [1]

Results from a retrospective study of 66,106 hospitalized adult neutropenic cancer patients showed that 2.7% to 12.1% of these patients experienced VTE during their first hospitalization. [2]

The association of VTE with underlying malignancy was first reported by Armand Trousseau in 1865, and the pathophysiologic explanations of the etiology of VTE in cancer include known hypercoagulability, vessel wall damage and vessel stasis from direct compression. Tumor cells can directly and indirectly promote the coagulation activation. They can stimulate the coagulation by producing tissue factors, expressing the coagulation factor X activator and by displaying surface sialic acid residues that can support non-enzymatic factor X activation.

They can also induce other cells, such as monocytes and endothelial cells, to elicit a tissue factor. Selected tumors may induce an accentuation of platelet activation and accumulation, whereas others tumors may express surface phospholipid species that support prothrombin and factor X activation. Cancer-related inflammation can result in increased concentrations of acute-phase proteins such as fibrinogen, factor VIII and the von Willebrand factor. Additional risk factors are: acquired or congenital thrombophilia, prolonged immobilization, use of drugs (chemotherapeutic regimens, selective oestrogen-receptor modulators, antiangiogenetic agents) and surgical procedures.

Clinical Presentation of VTE

VTE presentations include:

- Symptomatic deep vein thrombosis (DVT)
- Pulmonary embolism (PE)
- Superficial thrombophlebitis
- Central venous access device-associated thrombosis

Asymptomatic VTE can evolve into becoming symptomatic, and they may become particularly dangerous for the life of cancer patients.

Classical clinical symptoms of DVT are: pain, unilateral edema and heaviness in the distal extremity to the site of the venous thrombosis or edema in the face, neck or supraclavicular space. These signs and symptoms are not present in all cases so the diagnosis of DVT and PE made on clinical ground alone is notoriously unreliable. For example, the severity of limb edema, the presence of pain and dyspnoea are often unrelated to the location and extent of the thrombosis and depend on a patient's cardiopulmonary reserve. Symptoms can often be attributable to the underlying malignancy; however, it is important to be aware that VTE is a common complication of cancer to avoid missing a diagnosis of DVT or PE.

Table 1. Wells Clinical Deep Vein Thrombosis Model

Clinical characteristics	Score
Active cancer (pts receiving treatment for cancer within 6 months or currently receiving palliative care)	1
Paralysis, paresis or recent plaster cast immobilization of the lower extremities	1
Recent bedrest for 3 days or more, or major surgery within the previous 12 weeks requiring general or regional anesthesia	1
Localized tenderness along the distributionof the deep venous system	1
Entire leg swollen	1
Calf swelling at least 3 cm larger than the asymptomatic side (measured 10 cm below the tibial tuberosity)	1
Pitting edema confined to the symptomatic leg	1
Collateral superficial veins (non-varicose)	1
Previously documented deep vein thrombosis	1
Alternative diagnosis at least as likely as deep vein thrombosis	-2

Note: a score <2 indicates that DVT is unlikely.

Table 2. Wells Clinical Pulmonary Embolism Model

Clinical characteristics	Score
Active cancer (pts receiving treatment for cancer within 6 months or currently receiving palliative care)	1
Surgery or bedridden for 3 days or more during the past 4 weeks	1.5
History of DVT or PE	1.5
Hemoptysis	1
Heart rate>100 bpm	1.5
PE judged to be the most likely diagnosis	3
Clinical signs and symptoms compatible with DVT	3

The clinical Homans' sign, described as discomfort triggered by the passive dorsiflexion of the foot, is present in 8-60% of symptomatic patients with confirmed DVT and up to 40% of symptomatic persons without DVT. [3]

Particular features of the underlying malignancy could lead to a false-positive diagnosis of DVT or PE. Examples include the direct invasion or extrinsic vessel compression by a bulky tumor or adenopathy. The most widely used clinical prediction rules are the Wells DVT and PE models (Table 1 and 2), demonstrated to effectively rule out VTE in low-risk patients without using objective imaging studies. A low or unlikely score on the Wells CPR and a negative D-dimer result were associated with negative predictive values of 100% for both. [4-6] However, these studies included only a small number of subjects with cancer (9% to 14%); thus, these approaches are less rewarding in patients with cancer because few patients have a low probability of VTE and/or a negative D-dimer assay. [7]

Diagnosis of VTE

To ensure that patients are appropriately treated, VTE should be classified as:

1. Superficial versus deep
2. Distal versus proximal
3. Acute versus remote
4. Venous filling defect versus extrinsic vessel compression

A clinical suspicion for VTE in cancer patients requires sensitive imaging studies to assess for venous thrombus. The non-invasive imaging techniques available are a color duplex ultrasonography, spiral chest CT and ventilation-perfusion scan. In some cases, it could be useful to employ invasive imaging techniques such as CT or MR venography.

- Color duplex ultrasonography is the most appropriate initial diagnostic test, owing to the combination of accuracy, non-invasiveness, short examination time, portability of newer equipment and lower cost. It combines the real-time B mode ultrasound that provides the direct visualization of the vessels, with the pulsed-color Doppler flow imaging of red blood cells. The examination is based on vein wall compressibility, vein dilatation, visualization of echogenic intraluminal material and the spontaneous blood flow. Even if the specificity is always very high (89-100%), the sensibility varies on the location and extent of the thrombosis: the sensitivity of compression duplex ultrasound for acute femoro-popliteal DVT have been reported to be 92-100%, whereas it is lower in CVC-associated upper extremity DVT (82%) that tends to be more centrally located and for DVT above the inguinal ligament such as common iliac and proximal external iliac veins (62%). [8-10]
CT contrast venography is the imaging test of choice in this location. Right brachiocephalic veins and the superior vein cava are not usually visualized by the ultrasound and even if visualized, it is hard to make a diagnosis because of the incompressibility in these anatomical positions. DVT in this location is suggested by indirect Doppler-flow criteria, such as a lack of diameter change with inspiration and incomplete color filling of the lumen, and by the presence of echogenic intaluminal material with a B-mode ultrasound.
- The spiral chest CT is the primary imaging modality of diagnosis in PE. Criteria for acute DVT include a visualization of a filling defect in an opacified vein, a non-opacified segment between normally opacified proximal and distal segments, venous dilatation and venous wall ring enhancement. Sensitivity and specificity range from 53-100% and 78-100%, respectively. [3, 11] Advantages of a CT include the ability to visualize thoracic veins and concomitant extrinsic venous compression. False positives are possible because of flow artifacts, muscle hematomas and abscesses. [12]

- The ventilation-perfusion (V/Q) lung scan combines the inhalation of a radioactive gas (e.g. xenon), which provides an image of all ventilated areas of the lung, with a perfusion by intravenous injections of [Tc-99m]-labeled macroaggregated human serum albumin particles. Any obstruction to arterial flow is showed as a perfusion defect on gamma-camera images. According to the PIOPED criteria, on the basis of the presence and the extent of matched and unmatched defects of perfusion and ventilation, the V/Q scan can be interpreted as normal, low probability, intermediate or high probability for PE. A normal V-Q scan result essentially excludes PE. Both intermediate- and low-probability V-Q scan results lack diagnostic utility and should be considered indeterminate. In a patient clinically suspected to have PE, a high-probablility V-Q scan is diagnostic. Pleural effusions, chronic obstructive pulmonary disease, atelectasis, prior radiation to the chest and pulmonary masses and infiltrates are associated with a higher frequency of indeterminate-probability scans with a lower positive predictive value, whereas false high-probability scans may occur as a consequence of an abnormal perfusion scan due to a pulmonary artery invasion or compression, regional hypoventilation secondary to bronchial compromise, pulmonary vein obstruction by hilar mass or adenopathy, and pulmonary leukostasis. A V/Q scan should be reserved for patients with contrasting allergies or renal insufficiency because it doesn't employ iodinated contrast, and in pregnant patients in whom pulmonary scintigraphy probably results in fractionally lower fatal radiation doses compared with spiral CT angiography. [13]
- CT or MR venography, once considered the gold standard, has now been replaced by less invasive methods. Popliteal, or common femoral vein access, is the most frequent access but, in some circumstances, it might be necessary to gain access through an internal jugular vein. It could be important for diagnosising venous thrombosis in areas poorly visualized by the duplex ultrasound (thorax, abdomen, cerebral vasculature), providing information about surrounding structures, but it should be noticed that not all intraluminal filling defects represent thrombus in cancer patients, and the differential diagnosis might require further investigation with a CT or MRI. [14]
- D-dimer (semiquantitative and quantitative testing) is a degradation product of cross-linked fibrin and high levels of D-dimer and

prothrombin fragments 1 and 2 (F1+2), indicating a global coagulation activation and fibrinolysis, and has been reported in patients with malignancies in the absence of VTE. [15-18] For this reason, D-dimer testing is likely less sensitive and less specific in cancer patients, producing a high false-positive rate and a very low positive predictive value for thrombosis. Elevated levels of D-dimer and F1+2 most probably reflect a state of hypercoagulability which could be influenced by anticoagulation. A recent, large prospective study showed that elevated levels of D-dimer and F1+2 were independently associated with an increased risk for VTE occurrence. A detailed analysis revealed that patients with cancer who had both elevated D-dimer and elevated F1+2 had the highest risk of developing VTE (3.6-fold increased risk). [19] Elevated D-dimer levels have also been shown to be predictive of recurrent VTE in patients with cancer. [20] Conversely, a negative D-dimer test, when there is a low likelihood of VTE, can be used to effectively rule out a DVT diagnosis, although this combination rarely occurs in patients with cancer. [21, 22]

Risk Factors for VTE

This data about hypercoagulability in cancer patients is important not only to understand the mechanisms of cancer-associated VTE, but also to identify patients at high risk for VTE that could benefit from prophylactic anticoagulation treatment.

A risk-scoring model for chemotherapy-associated thrombosis, incorporating clinical and laboratory parameters (site of cancer, platelet count, haemoglobin and/or use of erythropoiesis-stimulating agents, leukocyte count and body mass index) (Table 3-4), was developed to define high-risk patients and to predict VTE in the ambulatory setting. At the cut-off point for high risk (score ≥3), the model had a negative predictive value of 98.5%. [23] This risk assessment model has been recently validated and extended by Ay et al. [24] who identified D-dimer and P-selectin as additional discriminatory risk factors. However, these laboratory tests are not routinely measured in cancer patients; they set stage for prospective confirmatory randomized clinical trials that evaluate the risk-benefit of VTE prophylaxis.

An Italian prospective trial in patients with breast cancer and gastro-intestinal (GI) cancer, receiving adjuvant chemotherapy, showed that the incidence of VTE during the treatment was 7.35%, whereas it was 0.52% during the subsequent follow-up. A multivariate analysis showed that thrombocytosis (PLT$\geq$ 300.000/mmc) and a history of thrombosis are risk factors for developing a thrombotic event in patients with malignant disease. [1-6, 25] The risk of VTE also depends on the chemotherapy regimens employed. Chemotherapy is recognized as an independent risk factor for thrombosis and may cause damage to the vascular endothelium, disequilibrium between procoagulant and anticoagulant molecules, tumor/endothelial apoptosis, cytokines activation and increased factor acitivity.

A prospective analysis quantified the incidence of thromboembolism among patients with advanced gastroesophageal cancer who were treated with four different triplet regimens (epirubicin, cisplatin, fluorouracil [ECF], epirubicin, cisplatin, capecitabine [ECX], epirubucun, fluorouracil, oxaliplatin [EOF] and epirubicin, oxaliplatin, capecitabine [EOX]). The study showed a different thrombogenic effect according to platinum use. [26]

The incidence of any TEs among 964 patients treated was 12.1%: it was more venous (10.1%) than arterial (2.2%). There was no significant difference in the overall incidence of TEs between fluorouracil and capecitabine, whereas there were fewer TEs in the oxaliplatin compared with cisplatin groups (EOF/EOX vs ECF/ECX: 7.6% vs 15.1%; p=.0003). Cisplatin was identified as a risk factor for TE in a multivariate analysis (HR=0.51; 95% CI, 0.34 to 0.76; p=.001). Potential mechanisms for cisplatin-associated vascular toxicity include hypomagnesemia, direct damage to the endovasculature and elevated von Willebrand factor.

The anti-vascular endothelial growth factor agent bevacizumab has also been associated with an increased risk of VTE in one meta-analysis [27]. Another analysis found no increased risk of VTE in patients treated with bevacizumab [28], but found an increasing risk of arterial thromboembolisms (ATEs) from approximately 1% to 3%.

Recently, another large pooled analysis, based on 6,055 patients, confirmed that there is no statistically significant increase in the risk of VTE related to bevacizumab. [29]

Central venous catheters (CVCs) are also associated with an increased risk of thrombosis. CVCs are widely used in the care of patients with cancer to administer chemotherapy and supportive care (including hydration, pain control and nutrition), transfusion therapy and acquire blood samples.

Table 3. Risk scoring model for chemotherapy-associated thrombosis

Patient characteristic	Risk score
Site of cancer	
Very high risk (stomach, pancreas)	2
High risk (lung, lymphoma, gynaecologic, bladder,testicular)	1
Prechemotherapy platelet count≥350,000/mmc	1
Hb < 10g/dl or use of RBC growth factors	1
Prechemotherapy leukocyte count >11,000/mmc	1
Body mass index ≥ 35 Kg/mq	1

Table 4. Risk scoring and rates of VTE

Risk category	Rates of VTE
Low (score=0)	0.8%
Intermediate (score=1-2)	1.8%
High (score≥3)	7.1%

Catheter-associated TEs are commonly asymptomatic, and multiple factors are involved in the pathogenesis of these events such as vessel wall injury, as a result of catheter insertion, venous stasis and vessel occlusion. All of these can lead to the formation of a thrombus associated with the catheter which, in turn, can lead to the occlusion of a deep vein of the upper extremity. Patients with tumors in the mediastinum or chest are at additional risk of thrombosis because of direct effects of these tumors on venous flow. The type of catheter, its number of lumen, the material and the method and site of insertion can influence the risk of thrombosis. Infection of an indwelling catheter is also felt to increase this risk.

VTE Risk Factors in Cancer Patients

General Patients Risk Factors

1.   Active cancer
2.   Advanced stage of cancer
3.   Cancer types at high risk:

- Brain
- Pancreas
- Stomach
- Bladder
- Gynaecologic
- Lung
- Lymphoma
- Mieloproliferative neoplasm
- Kidney
- Metastatic cancers

4. Regional bulky limphoadenopathy with extrinsic vascular compression
5. Familial and/or acquired hypercoagulability (including pregnancy)
6. Medical comorbidities (infections, renal disease, pulmonary disease, congestive heart failure, arterial thromboembolism)
7. Poor performance status
8. Older age

Treatment-Related Risk Factors

- Major surgery
- Central venous catheter /IV catheter
- Chemotherapy (especially use of thalidomide/lenalidomide plus high dose dexamethasone)
- Exogenous estrogen compunds (hormone replacement, contraceptives, tamoxifen/raloxifen, diethylstilbestrol)

Modifiable Risk Factors

- Obesity
- Smoking/tobacco
- Activity exercise

Multiple Myeloma Risk Factors [30]

- M spike>1.6g/dl
- Progressive disease
- Hyperviscosity

Therapies for Prophylaxis or Treatment of VTE in Cancer Patients

The only placebo-controlled, randomized clinical trial associated with the use of anticoagulants to treat VTE was performed in 1960 [31-32]: patients with clinically diagnosed PE were randomly assigned to heparin and nicoumalone, or to no anticoagulation. Of the 16 patients assigned to anticoagulation therapy, there were no deaths compared with five deaths and five non-fatal recurrences in the 19 patients randomly assigned to no treatment. Most of the subsequent non-placebo-controlled clinical trials, evaluating the use of anticoagulant therapy in VTE, support the evidence that these treatments are very effective. The specific therapy and duration of treatment in cancer patients depends on the location of the thrombus (e.g., ilio-femoral DVT vs PE), treatment-related risk factors (e.g., thalidomide based therapy), extent of the thrombus (e.g., subsegmental PE versus massive PE) and patient comorbities (e.g., brain metastases). In general, it seems prudent to treat for a minimum of 6 months and at least until all cancer therapy has been completed or, if possible, there are no residual malignancies.

Cancer patients could have a propensity toward heparin resistance that can be related to a disseminated intravascular coagulation (DIC) or to the binding of heparin to mononuclear white cells, acute-phase proteins (histidine-rich protein, vitronectin and platelet factor 4) and vascular endothelial cells. Cancer patients can also manifest an "apparent" heparin resistance characterized by a dissociation between the value of aPTT, that is normal, and the level of heparin concentration. This phenomenon is caused by elevated levels of factor VIII that can shorten the aPTT without affecting the antithrombotic actions of the drug.

Patients with malignancy can also experience recurrent VTE during warfarin treatment, despite an apparently stable INR between 2.0 and 3.0 (warfarin failure) because of an insufficiency of this degree of anticoagulation to neutralize the sum of hypercoagulable stimuli in a patient. Patients with warfain failure can either be treated with UFH or LMWH until a higher intensity of oral anticoagulation (INR: 3.0-4.0) is attained, or be switched to primary long-term therapy with LMWH.

Currently available drugs for preventing VTE are vitamin K antagonists (VKA), such as warfarin; unfractioned heparin (UFH); and low molecular weight heparins (LMWHs). LMWHs have a longer half-life and better bioavailability than UFH, and they are less hemorrhagic. None of these agents are ideal for prophylaxis in ambulatory patients: UFH and LMWHs require daily subcutaneous injections;warfarin can be difficult to administer because of nausea and vomiting, poor nutrition and interactions with other medications; and it requires laboratory monitoring. New antithrombotic agents, such as oral IIa and Xa inhibitors, could be useful. Nonetheless, further studies are needed.

Treatment of DVT

Low-Molecular Weight Heparins

On the basis of level I evidence from randomized controlled trials, LMWH is the preferred initial and long-term anticoagulation for VTE in cancer patients. This recommendation is largely based on the CLOT trial and three other smaller open trials comparing different LMWH with VKA for the long-term treatment of cancer-associated thrombosis. In the CLOT trial [33], patients with acute VTEs were randomized to dalteparin (200 IU/Kg/day for 1 month, successively reduced to 75-80% for further 5 months) or coumarin. VTE recurrences were 9% versus 17%, respectively, and this produced a statistically significant relative risk reduction of 53% (HR=0.48; p=0.002) and an absolute risk reduction of 8%. There was not a significant difference in major bleeding rates between two arms.

The LITE trial [34] randomized 200 patients with acute VTE to the standard treatment (UFH followed by warfarin with INR between 2 and 3, or initial and chronic anticoagulation with tinzaparin (175 IU/Kg/day). After 3 months, patients considered to be at risk for recurrent VTE continued warfarin (in the standard treatment arm) or initiated warfarin (if in LMWH arm). After 1 year, 16% of patients in the standard treatment arm and 7% in the LMWH arm experienced a recurrent VTE (p=0.044). There was no significant difference in bleeding in the two arms. Two other studies showed a consistent, but not statistically significant, benefit with LMWH over warfarin [35-36]: in the first one, enoxaparin 1.5 mg/Kg once a day was compared with warfarin given for 3 months in 146 patients with DVT and cancer. The study showed an increased rate of major outcome events, defined as major bleeding or recurrent VTE within 3 months, in the warfarin arm (21.1 vs. 10.5% p=0.09).

The Deitcher study [36] evaluated enoxaparin alone versus initial enoxaparin followed by warfarin for the secondary prevention of VTE in 122 adults with active malignancy. There were no significant differences in major and minor bleeding rates between treatment groups.

The major advantage of subcutaneous LMWH is that can be self-administered at home, without the need for therapeutic monitoring and lowers the risk of heparin-induced thrombocytopenia (HIT syndrome). This is an immunoglobulin-mediated serious complication of heparin therapy characterized by thrombocytopenia and is high risk for venous and arterial thrombosis. Two distinct types of HIT can occur: non-immune and immune-mediated HIT. Non-immune HIT, which occurs more frequently, is characterized by a mild decrease in the platelet count and is not harmful. The second type, immune-mediated HIT, occurs much less frequently but is dangerous. Immune-mediated HIT causes much lower platelet counts. Paradoxically, despite a very low platelet count, patients who suffer from HIT are at risk for major clotting problems. Immune-mediated HIT usually occurs from 5 to 14 days after first beginning heparin therapy. The condition of HIT is caused by antibodies, most frequently IgG, binding to the heparin–PF4 complex. The heparin–PF4 antibodies (sometimes called "HIT antibodies"), in the resultant multimolecular immune complex, activate platelets via their Fc receptors, causing the release of prothrombotic platelet-derived microparticles, platelet consumption, and thrombocytopenia [37]. The microparticles in turn promote excessive thrombin generation, frequently resulting in thrombosis. The antibody–antigen complexes also interact with monocytes, leading to tissue factor production. Thus, antibody-mediated endothelial injury may occur. Both of these latter processes may contribute further to thrombosis [37].

For patients who are receiving heparin or have received heparin within the previous 2 weeks, the American College of Chest Physicians Evidence-Based Clinical Practice Guidelines recommend investigating for a diagnosis of HIT if the platelet count falls by >50% and/or a thrombotic event occurs between days 5 and 14 (inclusive) following the initiation of heparin, even if the patient was no longer receiving heparin therapy when the thrombosis or thrombocytopenia occurred [38].

Warfarin

Warfarin is an option for long-term treatment of VTE in cancer patients, but it has a very narrow therapeutic window and its activity is known to be affected by poor nutrition, liver dysfunctions, GI disturbances and administration of many other drugs such as antibiotics and antifungal therapies (eg trimethoprim-sulfamethoxazole, ciprofloxacin, metronidazole and fluconazole) potentiate the effect of warfarin, whereas rifampin and dicloxacillin antagonize its effect [39-40].

Furthermore, certain chemotherapeutic agents, such as the fluoropyrimidines (5-fluorouracil and capecitabine), increase the international normalized ratio (INR) in patients treated with warfarin anticoagulation [41-42].

The target therapeutic INR range is 2.0 to 3.0 for treating VTE, but the maintenance of this level can also be very difficult because of periodically discontinuing the drug due to invasive procedures or chemotherapy-induced thrombocytopenia.

Unfractionated Heparin (UFH)

Before the introduction of LMWH, the standard of care for the initial treatment of VTE was intravenously-administered UFH. The major limitations of this regimen is the need for hospitalization and frequent activated partial thromboplastin time (aPTT) monitoring, whereas its advantages are the rapid reversibility of the anticoagulant effects and its possibility to be administered to patients with advanced renal failure. A meta-analysis of several trials showed that LMWH is safer, more efficacious and associated with lower mortality rates than UFH [43].

Recently, a randomized, multicenter trial compared dalteparin with UFH in critically ill patients and it showed no significant between-group difference associated with the rate of proximal leg deep-vein thrombosis, which occurred in 5.1% of patients in the intensive care unit receiving dalteparin and in 5.8% of patients receiving UFH, whereas PE was significantly lower with dalteparin (1.3% versus 2.3%; HR=0.51, p=0.01). LMWH is also associated with a lower risk of HIT syndrome and osteoporosis.

Fondaparinux

It is a synthetic pentasaccharide, and it is the only specific factor Xa inhibitor approved by the FDA for the prophylaxis and treatment of VTE. It binds rapidly to antithrombin in the blood and introduces a conformational change in the molecule that increase its inhibitory effect against factor Xa by a factor of approximately 300.

Fondaparinux is administered by subcutaneous injections, and its advantages include its ability to eliminate the need to monitor anticoagulant responses in most patients and its lack of cross-reactivity with the antibody associated with HIT syndrome [44-45, 38]. As reported by Turpie [46], the efficacy and safety of fondaparinux for postoperatively preventing thrombosis was studied in four trials and a meta-analysis of the latter, including 7,344 patients. The incidence of VTE was reduced from 13.7% with LMWH to 6.8% with fondaparinux (p<0.001). The corresponding rates of major bleeding were 1.7% and 2.7% respectively (p=0.008).

There has been one trial associated with the use of fondaparinux in patients with acute DVT and one trial in patients with acute PE [47-49]. Fondaparinux was equivalent to 1 week of LMWH followed by a long-term VKA.Only 10% of participants had cancer in these trials.

Fondaparinux has renal elimination, a very long half-time of 17-21 hours and there is no antidote. It is contraindicated in patients with severe renal failure (Ccr < 30 ml/min), weighing less than 50 Kg, and undergoing orthopaedic or abdominal surgery. It should be used with caution on elderly patients.

Other orally active factor Xa inhibitors, with no need of laboratory monitoring, are now being studied to investigate their efficacy in the prevention and treatment of VTE. Recently, an open-label, randomized study showed the non-inferiority of one of these, rivaroxaban, compared with subcutaneous enoxaparin followed by a vitamin K antagonist in patients with acute symptomatic DVT.

However, the proportion of patients with active cancer at the time of enrolment was only 7%. Thus, although both the relative efficacy and safety of rivaroxaban were similar to those of standard therapy in these patients, more data is needed [49].

Prophylactic Anticoagulation Therapy

The concept of thromboprophylaxis has been widely accepted in primarily the surgical setting for more than 25 years, but only in the last decade has thst acceptance spread to the widespread application associated with cancer patients. The risks and the advantages from prophylactic therapy should be considered as well and, on the basis of current data, we should differentiate indications to therapy in hospitalized and ambulatory patients.

1) Inpatients Prophylactic Therapy

Randomized clinical trials of prophylaxis for VTE, restricted specifically to patients with cancer, are unavailable and information regarding benefits and risks must be inferred from studies in surgical or general medical patients. Three large, randomized double-blind, placebo-controlled trials (MEDENOX, PREVENT and ARTEMIS trials) have demonstrated the benefits of anticoagulant prophylaxis in general medical patients [50-52], employing enoxaparin, dalteparin and fondaparinux respectively. Taken together, they clearly demonstrate that primary prophylaxis reduces VTE in hospitalized medical patients. Unfortunately, it should be noted that all of the studies include a heterogeneous population of medical patients in whom those with cancer represent a minority. Thus, in the PREVENT, MEDENOX and ARTEMIS studies, patients with cancer represented 5.1%, 12.4% and 15.4% of the total study groups respectively. However a subgroup analysis of the MEDENOX study showed that patients with cancer had an elevated risk of venous thromboembolisms and that the relative risk reduction for VTE in patients with cancer treated with enoxaparin was 0.50, similar to the benefits observed in the whole group.

Hospitalized patients with cancer are at high risk of VTE so, in abstention of contraindication, they should have prophylactic anticoagulation therapy.

2) Outpatients Prophylactic Therapy

Little data is available for ambulatory patients with cancer; thus, clinical trials are required before any recommendations can be made about this argument.

Although there is a lack of consistent evidence to support extended outpatient prophylaxis, it is recommended for multiple myeloma patients receiving high thrombogenic chemotherapy regimens (eg. thalidomide/lenalidomide plus high-dose dexamethasone). Two studies showed warfarin/LMWH prophylaxis were effective at reducing the risk of thromboembolisms in patients with advanced breast cancer receiving chemotherapy [53] and with advanced lung cancer [54].

The PROTECHT study (PROphylaxis of ThromboEmbolism during CHemotherapy), a randomized, placebo-controlled trial showed the efficacy of nadroparin (3800 IU/sc/day up to a maximum of 4 months) for the prophylaxis of thromboembolic events in ambulatory patients receiving chemotherapy for metastatic or locally advanced solid cancer: 2% of patients treated with nadroparin and 3.9% of patients in a placebo-arm experienced symptomatic thromboembolic events without a statistically significant risk of bleeding [55].

The PRODIGE trial evaluated LMWH prophylaxis in patients with malignant brain tumors. In this study, patients with newly diagnosed grade 3 or 4 glioma were randomly allocated to receive either dalteparin or placebo, both administered subcutaneously for 6 months. Ninety-nine patients received dalteparin and 87 received placebo; 9 LMWH patients experienced VTE compared with 13 placebo patients (HR=0.6) with 5 major bleeding in the LMWH arm and one in the placebo arm [56].

Recently, the SAVE-ONCO study, a randomized double-blind multicenter trial, showed the efficacy and the safety of the ultra-low molecular weight heparin semuloparin for preventing a nous thromboembolism in patients receiving chemotherapy for locally advanced or metastatic solid tumors. Semuloparin reduced the incidence of the thromboembolic events in a statistically significant manner (3.4% vs 1.2%, HR=0.36, p<0.001) with no apparent increase in major bleeding [57].

Prophylactic Anticoagulation Therapy Contraindications to Prophylactic/ Therapeutic Anticoagulation Treatment

The use of anticoagulant drugs in cancer patients is complicated by the fact that these patients have higher risks of both recurrent VTE and bleeding. In some circumstances, the use of these agents is temporary or permanently contraindicated. Contraindications could include:

- Clinically significant active or chronic bleeding
- Recent central nervous system bleeding or intracranial or spinal lesions at high risk for bleeding
- Spinal anesthesia/ lumbar puncture
- Patients at high risk for falls and/or head trauma
- Thrombocytopenia or platelets dysfunctions
- Systemic coagulopathy

Placing an inferior vena cava (IVC) filter is an option in cancer patients with acute VTE and an unacceptable bleeding risk or major bleeding complications during anticoagulation therapy. However, we can't forget that IVC is thrombogenic and anticoagulation therapy should start or resume if the acute bleeding risk factors resolve.

Indications for thrombolytic therapy are limited to PE, causing a severe hemodynamic instability, or a DVT causing arterial insufficiency in the affected limb due to severe venous congestion and CVC occlusion. In other cases, the thrombolytic therapy should be avoided because of the increased risk of bleeding, especially in patients with brain metastases.

Other limitations to IVC filters include technical difficulties during insertion, obstructions below the filter, filter migration or tilting, caval erosion and perforation, and filter failure.

Future Prospects

It is clear the importance of thrombosis in patients with malignancy, and oncologists should pay attention to early diagnosis, prophylactic treatment and the acute and chronic management of VTE. Although there continues to be improvements, some questions remain open such as the efficacy and safety of treatment of VTE with LMWH beyond 6 months, the long-term surveillance of cancer patients, the treatment on incidental thrombosis (whether all patients or only a subset be treated), and treatment in pregnant patients with cancer or patients with primary/secondary brain tumors.

Also interesting is the development of new oral drugs that do not have the narrow window of warfarin and that could make long-term anticoagulation more appealing to all patient populations. Ongoing research, evaluating the link between thrombosis and accelerated tumor neovascularisation, growth and metastases, may highlight the importance of thrombosis prevention in all cancer patients.

We hope that future clinical trials further address these notions and that they will help to optimize the care of cancer patients at risk or affected by VTE.

References

[1] Lyman GH, Khoarana AA, Falnga A, et al. American Society of Clinical Oncology guidelines: recommendations for venous thromboembolism prophylaxis and treatment in patients with cancer. *J. Clin. Oncol.* 2007; 25: 5490-5505.

[2] Korana AA, Francis CW, Culakova E et al. Thromboembolism in hospitalized neutropenic cancer patients. *J. Clin. Oncol.* 2006; 24: 484-90.

[3] Gomes MPV, Deitcher SR. Diagnosis of venous thromboembolic disease in cancer patients. *Oncology.* 2003; 17: 126-35.

[4] Kearon C, Ginsberg JS, Douketis J et al. An evaluation of D-dimer in the diagnosis of pulmonary embolism: a randomized trial. *Ann. Intern. Med.* 2006; 144: 812-821.

[5] Wells PS, Anderson DR, Rodger M et al. Evaluation of D-dimer in the diagnosis of suspected deep-vein thrombosis *N. Engl. J. Med.* 2003; 349: 1227-35.

[6] Van Belle A, Buller HR, Huisman MV et al. Effectiveness of managing suspected pulmonary embolism using an algorithm combining clinical probability, D-dimer, and computed tomography. *JAMA.* 2006; 295: 172-9.

[7] Carrier M, Lee Ay, Bates Sm et al. Accuracy and usefulness of a clinical prediction rule and d-dimer testing in excluding deep vein thrombosis in cancer patients. *Thromb. Res.* 2008; 123: 177-83.

[8] Kearon C, Julian JA, Newman TE et al. Non-invasive diagnosis of deep venous thrombosis *Ann. Intern. Med.* 1998; 128: 663-77.

[9] Baarslag HJ, van Beek EJ, Koopman MM et al. Prospective study of color duplex ultrasonography compared with contrast venography in patients suspected of having deep vein thrombosis of the upper extremitics. *Ann. Intern. Med.* 2002; 136: 865-72.

[10] Rosovsky RP, Kuter DJ. Catheter-related thrombosis in cancer patients: pathophysiology, diagnosis and management. *Henatol. Oncol. Clin. North Am.* 2005; 19: 183-202.

[11] Deitcher SR, Carman TL. Deep venous thrombosis and pulmonary embolism. *Curr. Treat. Options Cardiovasc. Med.* 2002; 4: 223-38.

[12] Gaye B, Szapiro D, Willems V, et al. Pitfalls in CT venography of lower limbs and abdominal veins. *AJR. Am. J. Roentgenol.* 2002; 178: 1465-71.

[13] Stein PD, Wooddard PK, Weg JG et al. Diagnostic pathways in acute pulmonary embolism: recommendations of the PIOPED II investigatots. *Radiology.* 2007; 242:15-21.

[14] Rosovsky RP, Kuter DJ. Catheter-related thrombosis in cancer patients: pathophysiology, diagnosis and management. *Henatol. Oncol. Clin. North. Am.* 2005; 19: 183-202.

[15] Kohli M, Fink LM; Spencer HJ et al. Advanced prostate cancer activates coagulation. A controlled study of activation markers of coagulation in ambulatory patients with localized advanced prostate cancer. *Blood Coagul. Fibrinolysis.* 2002; 13:1-5.

[16] Hanzal E. Tatra G. Prothrombin fragment F1+2 plasma concentrations in patients with gynaecologic malignancies. *Gynecol. Oncol.* 1993; 49: 373-6.

[17] Lippi G, Franchini M, Targher G et al. Help me doctor! My D-dimer is raised. *Ann. Med.* 2008; 40: 594-605.

[18] Seitz R, Rappe N, Kraus M et al. Activation of coagulation and fibrinolysis in patients with lung cancer: relation to tumor stage and prognosis. *Blood Coagul. Fibrinolysis.* 1993; 4: 249-54.

[19] Cihan Ay, Vormittang R, Dunkler D et al. D-dimer and prothrombin fragment 1+2 predict venous thromboembolism in patients with cancer: results from the Vienna Cancer and thrombosis study. *J. Clin. Oncol.* 2009; 25: 4124-9.

[20] Sallah S, Husain A, Sigounas V et al. Plasma coagulation markers in patients with solid tumors and venous thromboembolic disease receiving oral anticoagulation therapy. *Clin. Cancer Res.* 2004; 10: 7238-43.

[21] Ten Wolde M, Kraaijenhagen RA, Prins Mh et al. The clinical usefulness of D-dimer testing in cancer patients with suspected deep venous thrombosis. *Arch. Intern. Med.* 2002; 162: 1880-4.

[22] Carrier M, Lee Ay, Bates SM et al. Accuracy and usefulness of a clinical prediction rule and D-dimer testing in excluding deep vein thrombosis in cancer patients. *Thromb. Res.* 2008; 123: 177-83.

[23] Khorana AA, Kuderer NM, Culakova E et al. Development and validation of a predictive model for chemotherapy-associated thrombosis. *Blood.* 2008; 111: 4902-7.

[24] Ay C, Dunkler D, Marosi C et al. Prediction of venous thromboembolism in cancer patients. *Blood.* 2010; 116; 5377-82.

[25] Mandalà M, Barni S, Prins M et al. Acquired and inherited risk factors for developing venous thromboembolism in cancer patients receiving adjuvant chemotherapy: a prospective trial. *Ann. Oncol.* 2010; 21: 871-6.

[26] Straling N, Rao S, Cunningham D et al. Thromboembolism in patients with advanced gastroesophageal cancer treated with anthracycline, platinum and fluoropyrimidine combination chemotherapy: a report from the UK National Cancer Research Institute Upper Gastrointestinal Clinical Studies Group. *J. Clin. Oncol.* 2009; 23: 3786-93.

[27] Nalluri SR, Chu D, Keresztes R et al. Risk of venous thromboembolism with the angiogenesis inhibitor bevacizumab in cancer patients: a metanalysis. *JAMA.* 2008; 300: 2277-85.

[28] Scappaticci FA, Skilling JR, Holden SN et al. Arterial thromboembolic events in patients with metastatic carcinoma treated with chemotherapy and bevacizumab. *J. Natl. Cancer Inst.* 2007; 99: 1232-9.

[29] Hurwitz HI, Saltz LB, Van Cutsem E et al. Venous thromboembolic events with chemotherapy plus bevaciuzmab: a pooled analysis of patients in randomized phase II and III studies. *J. Clin. Oncol.* 2011; 29: 1757-64.

[30] Palumbo A, Rajkumar SV, Dimopoulos Ma, et al. Prevention of thalidomide- and lenalidomide-associated thombosis in myeoloma. *Leukemia.* 2008; 22: 414-23.

[31] Barrit DW, Jordan SC. Anticoagulant drugs in the treatment of pulmonary embolism. A controlled trial *Lancet.* 1960; 1: 1309-12.

[32] Hirsh J, Bates SM. Clinical trials thet have influenced the treatment of venous thromboembolism:a historical perspective. *Ann. Intern. Med.* 2001; 134: 409-17.

[33] Samama MM, Cohen AT, Darmon J-Y et al. A comparison of enoxaparin with placebo for the prevention of venous thromboembolism in acutely ill medical patients. *N. Engl. J. Med.* 1999; 341: 793-800.

[34] Leizorovicz A, Cohen AT, Turpie AG et al. Randomized, placebo-controlled trial of dalteparin for the prevention of venous thromboembolism in acutely ill medical patients. *Circulation.* 2004; 110: 874-9.

[35] Cohen AT, Davidson BL, Gallus et al. Efficacy and safety of fondaparinux for the prevention of venous trhomboembolism in older acute medical patients: randomised placebo controlled trial. *BMJ.* 2006; 332: 325-9.

[36] Levine MN, Hirsh J, Gent M et al. Double-blind randomized trial of very-low-dose warfarin for the prevention of thromboembolism in stage IV breast cancer. *Lancet* 1994; 343: 886-9.

[37] Haas S. Prevention of venous thromboembolism with low-molecular-weight-heparin in patients with breast and lung cancer. Result of the TOPIC studies. *J. Thromb. Haemost.* 2005; 2(S1): abs OR059.

[38] Perry JR, Rogers L, Laperriere N et al. PRODIGE: a phase III randomized placebo-controlled trial of thromboprophylaxis using dalteparin low molecular weight heparin (LMWH) patients with newly diagnosed malignant glioma (JCO 2007; 25:77#2011.

[39] Lee A, Levine M, Baker RI et al Low-molecular-weight-heparin versus a Coumarin for the prevention of a recurrent venous thromboembolism in patients with cancer. *N. Engl. J. Med.* 2003; 349: 146-53.

[40] Hull R, Pineo G, Brant RF et al. Long term low-molecular-weight-heparin versus usual care in proximal-vein thrombosis patients with cancer *Am. J. Med.* 2006; 119: 1062-72.

[41] Meyer G, Marjanovic Z, Valcke J et al. Comparison of low-molecular-weight-heparin and warfarin for the secondary prevention of venous thromboembolism in patients with cancer: a randomized controlled study. *Arch. Intern. Med.* 2002; 162: 1729-35.

[42] Deithcher SR, Kessler CM, Merli G et al. Secondary prevention of venous thromboembolic events in patients with active cancer: enoxaparin alone versus initial enoxaparin followed by warfarin for a 180-day period. *Clin. Appl. Thromb. Hemost.* 2006; 12: 389-96.

[43] Aronson J. Serious drug interactions. *Practitioner.* 1993; 237:789-791.

[44] Lacey CS. Interactions of dicloxacillin with warfarin. *Ann. Pharmacother.* 2004; 38: 898.

[45] Saif MW. An adverse interaction between warfarin and fluoropyrimidnes revisited. *Clin. Colorectal. Cancer.* 2005; 5: 175-80.

[46] Shah HR, Ledbetter L, Diasio R et al. A retrospective study of coagulation abnormalities in patients receiving capecitabine and warfarin. *Clin. Colorectal. Cancer.* 2006; 5: 354-8.

[47] van Dongen CJ, van den Belt AG, Prins MH et al. Fixed dose subcutaneous low molecular weight heparins versus adjusted dose

unfractionated heparin for venous thromboembolism. *Cochrane Database Sys. Rev.* 2004.

[48] Glaxo Smith Kline. Prescribing information: Arixtra (fondaparinux).

[49] Prandoni P. How I treat venous thromboembolism in patients with cancer. *Blood.* 2005; 106: 4027-33.

[50] Warkentin TE, Greinacher A et al. Effect of fondaparinux on platelet activation in the presence of heparin-dependent antibodies: a blinded comparative multicenter study with unfractionated heparin. *Chest* 2008; 133: 340S-80S.

[51] Turpie AGG, Bauer KA, Eriksson BI et al. Fondaparinux vs enoxaparin for the prevention of venous thromboembolism after hip-fracture surgery. *Arch. Intern. Med.* 2002; 162: 1833-40.

[52] Buller HR, Davidson BL, Decousus H et al. Subcutaneous fondaparinux versus intravenous unfractionated heparin in the initial treatment of pulmonary embolism. *N. Engl. J. Med.* 2003; 349: 1695-1702.

[53] Buller HR, Davidson BL, Decousus H et al. Fondaparinux or enoxaparin for the initial treatment of symptomatic deep venous thrombosis: a randomized trial. *Ann. Intern. Med.* 2004; 140: 867-873.

[54] Landman GW, Gans RO. Oral rivaroxaban for symptomatic venous thromboembolism. *N. Engl. J. Med.* 2011; 364: 1178.

[55] Jang IK, Hursting MJ. When heparins promote thrombosis: review of heparin-induced thrombocytopenia. *Circulation.* 2005; 111: 2671-83.

[56] The PROTECT investigators for the Canadian critical care trials group and the Australian and the New Zealand intensive care society clinical trails group. Dalteparin versus unfractionated heparin in critically ill patients. *N. Eng. J. Med.* 2011; 364:1305-1314.

[57] Agnelli G, George D, Ajay K et al. Semuloparin for thromboprophylaxis in patients receiving chemotherapy for cancer. *N. Engl. J. M.* 2012; 366:601-609.

In: Deep Vein Thrombosis
Editor: Takashi Yamaki

ISBN: 978-1-62257-519-0
© 2013 Nova Science Publishers, Inc.

Chapter 3

Prevention of Deep Vein Thrombosis in Neurological Surgery

Mario Ganau[*] *and Leonello Tacconi*
Department of Neurosurgery, University Hospital Trieste, Trieste, Italy

Abstract

Background: The mean incidence of deep vein thrombosis (DVT) in neurosurgical reports is variable and surprisingly approaches 25%, whereas the incidence of pulmonary embolism (PE) is thought to be between 1.5% and 3%, with a mortality rate between 9% and 50%. Although DVT is probably the single most important, preventable cause of morbidity and mortality in this domain, its pharmacologic prevention is still a controversial matter due to the concern associated with the possible increased risk of postoperative haemorrhaging. Prophylactic options against DVT/PE include elastic stockings, intermittent pneumatic compression devices, low-dose unfractionated heparin (UFH), and low molecular-weight heparin (LMWH). The aim of this chapter is to describe the prophylactic protocols for DVT currently in use in neurological surgery and share our experience on this topic.

[*] Correspondence to: Mario Ganau MD, MSBM. Neurosurgery, University Hospital Trieste, Strada di Fiume 447-34149 Trieste, ITALY. TEL: +39-040-399-4735. FAX: +39-040-399-4057. E-mail: mario.ganau@aots.sanita.fvg.it.

Analysis of the prophylactic protocols in neurological surgery: Systematic reviews of the English literature concerning DVT prophylactic protocols in neurosurgery have been conducted by a PubMed search (back to 1986). at the latter aimed to analyze the risks and benefits associated with different prophylactic regimens: abstracts of all identified articles were reviewed, and detailed information from eligible articles was extracted.

Description of our own protocol: Herein, we describe the DVT prophylactic protocol currently in use at the Neurosurgical Department in Trieste (Italy) and report the related results obtained on more than 3,818 consecutive patients that have undergone neurosurgical cranial or spinal procedures at our institution since January 2004. All patients were screened with preoperative blood coagulation tests.According to the presence of risk factors in the anamnesis, the type of surgical procedure (minor or major cranial or spinal procedures) and expectations associated with their postoperative course (prolonged immobilization), the patients were then stratified into three classes of risk: low-, moderate- or high-risk subgroups. The protocol is associated with both pharmacological and mechanical prophylactic measures: administering LMWH (2,000 UI to 4,000 UI per day), elasting stockings and mechanical pneumatic sequential compression leg devices. The end points of this protocol are to keep the incidence of DVT, PE and postoperative haemorrhaging as low as possible. Over the years, they were assessed as follows: in the case of neurological deterioration, significant bleeding in the surgical site was promptly ruled out by a head or spinal CT scan, as well in the case of a clinical suspicion for DVT or PE, a duplex ultrasonography and a chest x-ray plus a perfusion CT scan were respectively performed.

Results: Although literature confirms that intermittent pneumatic compression devices provide an adequate reduction of DVT/PE in some cranial and combined cranial/spinal series, UFH or LMWH have proved to further reduce the incidence of PE, and partially reduce the incidence of DVT. Nevertheless, UFH-based prophylaxis showed a higher incidence of postoperative haemorrhaging (2% - 4% in cranial series, and 1% in spinal ones), whereas LMWH protocols present less bleeding drawbacks. Our prophylactic protocol was well tolerated in all patients; particularly the stratification of risk and subdivision into risk groups gave us the opportunity to avoid concerns regarding overtreatment. Clinical evidence of DVT occurred in 0.4% of our cohort; one patient died of fatal PE 2 months after surgery. Less than 1% of our patients presented significant postoperative haemorrhaging, mostly after major cranial surgery.

Conclusion: The results reported in literature confirm the need for a DVT prophylactic protocol in neurosurgical patients: a combined mechanical/pharmacological regimen seems to be the most appropriate and effective, but a prospective randomized trial to assess the best dosage, molecule and timing of LMWH administration is still lacking. On the other hand, even if our database only allows for an observational analysis, the results obtained in such a large group of neurosurgical patients are encouraging, since they show the efficacy in terms of DVT and PE prevention, without significant incidence of postoperative complications such as surgical-site haemorrhaging. Certainly, this data gives enough evidence to support the DVT prophylactic protocol applied throughout the last 6 years at our institution.

Introduction

The mean incidence of deep vein thrombosis (DVT) in neurosurgical reports is variable and surprisingly approaches 25%, whereas the incidence of pulmonary embolism (PE) is thought to be between 1.5% and 3%. Analyses of the major trials indicate that pulmonary embolisms are a major cause of death in neurosurgical patients with a mortality rate between 9% and 50%. [1, 2, 6, 8]

Fewer than one-third of patients with DVT will present with classic symptoms and signs such as a painful, swollen, and erythematous extremities; therefore, the different sensitivities of diagnostic measures may explain the different percentages of incidences reported in the literature for clinically overt and objectively-proven DVT. The first one has been reported to range from 1.6% to 4%, the second has been estimated to range from 19% to 43% in case series using fibrinogen labelled with iodine 125 (I^{125}) as the screening tool of choice, and from 24% to 33% in clinical trials using venography to screen for DVT. [1]

During prolonged general anaesthesia or any other period of limited mobility, a thrombus formation may be initiated in the deep veins of the leg. Such thrombosis is precipitated by the presence, to varying degrees, of components associated with Virchow's triad of risk factors (damage to the venous wall, change in blood flow and hypercoagulability). Venous stasis of the lower limbs is a consequence of immobility, whereas hypercoagulability may be secondary to tissue damage, inflammation or malignant disease. In neurosurgical patients, an intrinsic degree of hypercoagulability may be related to the relapse in fibropeptide A, fibrinogen, factor VIII and thromboplastin determined by brain tumors, brain or vertebral traumas, and even brain manipulation during surgical procedures.

Among neurosurgical patients, higher-risk subgroups for developing DVT may be identified according to the presence of one or more of the following criteria in the anamnesis: preoperative bed rest, obesity, oral contraceptives, previous episode of DVT and/or PE, severe neurological deficits such as dense hemiparesis or hemiplegia; as well as in case of the following operative criteria: presence of metastatic disease or malignancy, large size meningioma (diameter larger than 6 cm), expectation of a prolonged operation (more than 4 hours), and/or postoperative bed rest (more than 72 hours). Those with genetic hypercoagulopathic syndromes, including the factor V Leiden mutation; elevated antiphospholipid antibodies; and deficiencies of antithrombin, protein C, and protein S are also uniquely susceptible to new-onset and/or recurrent DVT and PE after neurosurgical procedures. [2]

Gallus et al. looked into and provided the estimates of the expected incidence of thromboembolic events in unprophylaxed patients. According to the abovementioned classification, moderate-risk patients presented the expected incidence of calf (distal) DVT of 10%-40%, proximal DVT of 2%-8%, symptomatic pulmonary emboli of 1%-8% and fatal pulmonary emboli of 0.1%-0.4%. Patients at high risk have an expected incidence of distal DVT of 40%- 80%, proximal DVT of 10%-20%, symptomatic PE of 5%-10% and fatal PE of 1%-5%. Patients at low risk, presented an expected incidence of distal DVT of 2%, proximal DVT of 0.4%, symptomatic PE of 0.2% and fatal PE of 0.002%. [3]

Although DVT is probably the single most important, preventable cause of morbidity and mortality in this domain, its pharmacologic prevention is still a controversial matter due to the concern associated with the possible increased risk of postoperative haemorrhaging. Prophylaxis against DVT/PE is a critical issue, and options include: elastic stockings, intermittent pneumatic compression stockings, low-dose unfractionated heparin (UFH 5,000 U every 8-12 hours), and low molecular-weight heparin (LMWH, i.e., enoxaparin calcium and dalteparin sodium).

The aim of this chapter is to describe the prophylaxis protocols for DVT currently in use in neurological surgery and share our experience on this topic.

Analysis of the Prophylactic Protocols in the English Literature

Various mechanical and pharmacological methods of prophylaxis have been used to prevent DVT in high-risk patients, and numerous randomized controlled trials (RCTs) have been conducted among patients undergoing different neurosurgical procedures, and to a lesser extent among medical patients at high risk of DVT. To this regard, a systematic review of the literature concerning DVT prophylactic protocols in neurosurgery have been conducted by a PubMed search (back to 1978), 80 abstracts from all identified articles were reviewed, and detailed information from a total of eligible 69 articles [4-73] were extracted.

These analyses showed that, currently, most of the articles published in the literature on this subject are represented by case series and case reports; unfortunately, only a few of them are clinical trials dealing with standardized prophylactic protocols for DVT and PE.

Efficacy of Screening and Diagnostic Measures

Several studies have dealt with this topic, and the Doppler ultrasound is currently considered to be the most sensitive and specific test in detecting DVT with a negative predictive value of 97% - 98%. [31, 74] Noteworthy, Flinn et al. reported data on 2,643 patients undergoing cranial and spinal neurosurgical procedures in which Doppler studies were routinely performed 3 and 7 days after surgery and every week for the first few postoperative months. The routine Doppler screenings yielded more positive studies after cranial procedures as compared with spinal procedures. They concluded that craniotomies should routinely undergo ultrasound surveillance, whereas for patients undergoing spinal procedures, only those with a history of malignancy or paralysis should be routinely studied. [25]

On the other hand, an I^{125}-fibrinogen uptake test is based on the concept that the radioactive tracer is incorporated into actively forming thrombi. This technique is therefore insensitive in detecting thrombi that are not actively forming. [1]

The pulmonary angiography is the gold standard for segmental pulmonary embolisms (PE), but not for subsegmental PE. A normal perfusion lung scan and a normal rapid ELISA D-dimer test safely exclude PE. A helical spiral CT detects all clinically relevant PE and a large number of alternative diagnoses in symptomatic patients with a non-diagnostic ventilation perfusion scan (VP-scan) or a high probability VP-scan. A helical spiral CT can replace both the VP-scan and pulmonary angiography to safely rule PE in and out.

Michiels et al., in their recent paper concerning a critical appraisal of non-invasive diagnosing and exclusion testing for DVT and PE, reported that the negative predictive value of a normal helical spiral CT is 99% and that the combination of clinical assessment, a rapid ELISA D-dimer, followed by a Doppler ultrasound, will reduce the need for a helical spiral CT by 40% to 50%. [74]

Mechanical Compression

A comprehensive metanalysis on this topic, published in 2005 on Health Technology Assessments by Roderick et al. [75], concluded that mechanical compression methods may reduce the risk of DVT by about two-thirds when used as the only form of thromboprophylaxis, and by about half when added to a pharmacological method such as low-dose heparin. These benefits appear similar not only irrespective of the particular mechanical method used (e.g., intermittent pneumatic compression, graduated compression stocking and footpumps), but also similar in each of the surgical groups studied. [76] Mechanical methods appeared to reduce the risk of proximal DVT by about half, although this result may be subject to reporting bias since only a minority of trials reported proximal DVT as a specific outcome. [4, 14, 15] In their metanalysis, Roderick et al. showed that mechanical compression methods do not merely prevent the local consequences of leg thrombosis, but might also protect against more severe systemic embolic sequelae as an apparent reduction of about two-fifths in the risk of PE was found. [76]

The analyses of the literature clearly confirms that mechanical methods are effective even among patients who are already receiving a pharmacological method of thromboprophylaxis, such as low-dose heparin or aspirin, reducing the risk of DVT by about half in these circumstances. [9, 10, 11, 12, 24, 26, 53, 55] There are no uniform standards for providing DVT prophylaxis.

Chemoprophylaxis

A consensus statement published by the American College of Chest Physicians in 2001 indicated that intermittent pneumatic compression is the standard of care in all surgical patients and that UFH can be used at the discretion of the provider. [79]

The neurosurgical literature has documented a reduction in the incidence of DVT with heparin use, although concerns regarding the increased propensity for hemorrhaging have limited uniform and widespread applications associated with the drug. [5, 9, 18, 24, 26, 28, 41, 60, 65]

In fact, whereas mechanical prophylaxis with intermittent pneumatic compression used intraoperatively and postoperatively poses little to no risk in neurosurgical patients, problems attributed to hemorrhagic complications of low-dose subcutaneous UFH or LMWH regimens may prove devastating. [39]

In a neurosurgical series (cranial and spinal), the efficacy of mechanical compression alone or with low-dose subcutaneous UFH/LMWH prophylaxis was prospectively analyzed. Mechanical prophylaxis alone resulted in a 3.2% incidence of DVT and a 3.5% frequency of PE. IPC with low-dose subcutaneous UFH lowered the incidence of DVT/PE to 0%. [18] In patients who underwent craniotomies alone, MacDonald et al. similarly compared the results of prophylaxis with mechanical compression alone (68 patients refused to be included in the low-dose subcutaneous UFH group) with those obtained using both mechanical compression and low-dose subcutaneous UFH (5,000 U every 12 hours, 106 patients). For the nonheparin group, 4.4% (3 patients) of patients developed DVT, but 2.9% exhibited PE (1 fatal). For the low-dose subcutaneous UFH patients, the incidence of DVT was slightly higher, 6.6%, but the frequency of PE was lower at 0.94% (1 patient). Of note, the differences with the small number of patients included in these samples were not significant. [30]

However, the more widespread use of chemoprophylaxis is not without potential complications such as heparin-induced thrombocytopenia (HIT), which is an immune-mediated adverse drug reaction caused by the heparin-dependent platelet activation of IgG antibodies. Undoubtedly, the widespread application of heparin chemoprophylaxis in large numbers of patients will increase the prevalence of HIT. Although HIT is not well described in the neurosurgical literature, the reaction will have clear implications with the more extensive use of UFH.

Concluding, several systematic reviews of particular methods have been conducted, but the literature remains incomplete in some areas and contradictory in others. The experience drawn from the general surgery has affected recommendations on the use of chemoprophylaxis in divergent neurosurgical patient subgroups, which may have unexpected consequences. Thus, the risk-benefit ratio of current treatment protocols primarily based on non-neurosurgical patient populations has yet to be analyzed in a systematic fashion.

Prophylaxis in Spinal Trauma

In 2010, Ploumis et al. surveyed neurosurgeons and orthopedic surgeons from the North America Spinal Trauma Study Group in an attempt to understand current practices in the perioperative administration of thromboprophylaxis in spinal surgery. [70] According to the results reported, no prophylaxis or mechanical prophylactic measures were routinely used for Spinal Cord Injury (SCI) and non-SCI spinal fracture patients by 36 (77%) and 40 (85%) respondents, respectively. After surgery, pharmacologic prophylaxis is generally prescribed by 42 (91%) and 28 (62%) surgeons for SCI and non-SCI spinal fracture patients, respectively. A statistically significant tendency to use more intensive prophylactic measures for patients with SCI (χ^2 test 10.86; p < 0.01), as well as a statistically significant longer duration of proposed thromboprophylaxis (χ^2 test, 24.62; p < 0.001), were highlighted. Postoperative pharmacologic thromboprophylaxis for elective anterior thoracolumbar spine surgeries was reported by 23 (51%) of the respondents, whereas only 18 (40%) used pharmacological prophylaxis in elective posterior thoracolumbar spine cases. Nevertheless, spine complications from LMWH were reported by 22 (47%) surgeons, including fatal pulmonary embolisms by 19 (40%) surgeons.

Postoperative pharmacologic thromboprophylaxis is currently considered unnecessary in patients with cervical spine injuries without SCI; however, it is recommended for cervical spine traumas with SCI or anterior thoracolumbar procedures irrespective of SCI. Pharmacologic thromboprophylaxis should be started preoperatively as soon as possible in SCI cases or in cases with a surgical delay, and it is recommended to be administered for at least 3 months post-injury.

Prophylaxis in Head Trauma

Patients sustaining traumatic injuries are at high risk for the development of a venous thromboembolism. The reported incidence of DVT in trauma patients ranges from 20 to 90%; whereas the reported incidence of PE in trauma patients varies between 2.3 and 22%. [76] The aging population and the survival of more severely injured patients may suggest an increasing risk of thromboembolism in the head trauma patient population. Accordingly, there has been a general reluctance over the years to use anticoagulant prophylaxis for patients with a head injury who have suffered intracranial bleeding or for who intracranial surgery is needed.

This aspect has been analyzed by Cupitt [34] and Stephens et al. [23] through surveys from UK neurosurgical centers assessing the use of physical and pharmacological prophylactic methods against thromboembolisms. Both concluded that patients undergoing emergency neurosurgery are less likely to receive any form of prophylaxis. There have been few randomized prospective studies assessing methods of thromboembolism prophylaxis in trauma patients; therefore, controversy exists as to the optimal method of prophylaxis in this high-risk population, and contraindications arise from associated injuries which often limit the potential options for prophylaxis in patients with head and multiple organ traumas.

Currently, specific guidelines have been provided concerning neither the best prophylactic methods nor the time of administration in neurotrauma patients; therefore, those aspects are still a matter of debate and those patients are still subjectively managed.

Prophylaxis in Neurosurgical Oncology

The management of DVT prophylaxis in patients undergoing neurosurgical treatment for tumors requires balancing the risks of hemorrhaging and thrombosis. [17, 29, 38, 40] In their paper published in 2004, Smith et al. identified. from their neurosurgery databases, 2,779 discharges of patients with tumors; patients' admissions were relatively well matched for age, sex, duration of stay, and tumor type: those with intracranial tumors had a higher incidence of PE than those with spinal tumors. Smith et al. found a lower incidence of DVT in patients undergoing spinal procedures when LMWH was used judiciously; nevertheless, the incidence of PE in patients undergoing cranial procedures was lower in those managed with protocols not including prophylaxis with anticoagulating agents. [55] According to the case series analyzed, the only reachable final statement is that oncological patients are at a higher risk to develop DVT and PE, but no agreement on the best prophylaxis has been found.

From the review published by Tabori et al. the risk of clinically significant DVT in children with brain tumors may be exceedingly low as compared to adults. These findings set the stage for future evaluations in view of the prospective studies that were done in adults and the possible significant implications for the prevention and possible etiologies of the disease. [45]

Recommendations for Inferior Vena Cava Filter Placement as Prophylaxis against DVT/PE in Neurosurgery

In their review on this subject, Epstein et al. gave some indication for inferior vena cava filter placement in neurosurgical patients, stating that those with a history of DVT or PE undergoing prolonged procedures may be candidates for a prophylactic preoperative inferior vena cava (IVC) filter placement. [52]

The case series reported by Britt et al. [77] and Wong et al. [35] determined that inferior vena cava (IVC) filters constitute an important adjunct or alternative to heparin prophylaxis or full anticoagulation, particularly in postsurgical patients in whom the risk of heparin related hemorrhaging threatens neurological function. In 2003 Streiff et al. agreed with this statement. [78]

The Trieste Protocol, Analytical Description and Relevant Results

Considering that most DVT might begin during surgery, it appears sensible to start prophylaxis before surgery. However, Raabe et al. have shown that starting prophylaxis before surgery was associated with an increased risk of bleeding when compared with starting after surgery. Furthermore, Dickinson et al., during a prospective, randomized, unblinded trial comparing the pharmacologic DVT prevention before surgery with a mechanical compression device and a mechanical compression device alone, experienced a high bleeding rate (11%), and thus, the trial was interrupted.

Starting from these results, it has been assumed that postoperative prophylaxis could be a safer and reasonable concept in neurosurgery. As reported above, in recent years, LWMH has shown to be more effective in preventing DVT without relevant differences in postoperative bleeding; furthermore, this type of heparin has a longer duration of action and a greater bioavailability, making it more easily and safely adsorbed via the subcutaneous route. With this in mind, we have created our internal anti-DVT/PE protocol.

The DVT prophylactic protocol was applied to more than 3,818 consecutive patients, since January 2004, undergoing neurosurgical cranial or spinal procedures at our institution. All patients were screened with preoperative blood coagulation tests including PTT, prothrombin time, fibrinogen, antithrombin III and platelet count. According to the presence of risk factors in anamnesis, the type of surgical procedure (minor or major cranial or spinal procedures) and expectation of postoperative course (prolonged immobilization, and type of pathology), our patients were stratified into three classes of risk: low-, moderate- and high-risk subgroups.

Description of the Protocol

The protocol consisted of pharmacological and mechanical prophylactic measures: administration of LMWH (Tinzaparin Sodium, Enoxaparin Calcium and Dalteparin Sodium were progressively adopted over the years with a dosage ranging from 2,000 UI to 4,000 UI per day), elastic stockings and a mechanical pneumatic sequential compression leg device.

Patients younger than 40 years, with no anamnestical risk factors, undergoing minor surgical procedures (generally lasting less than 60 minutes). such as stereotactic or frameless biopsies, functional procedures for trigeminal neuralgia, evacuation of chronic subdural hematoma, ventriculoperitoneal shunt, external or endoscopic ventriculostomy, were considered as low risk patients and started a pharmacological prophylaxis, with low-molecular-weight heparine only in cases of prolonged postoperative bed rest (lasting more than 48 hours).

Patients were included in the moderate-risk subgroup in the following cases: age older than 40 years; minor or moderate brain traumas (Glasgow Coma Scale > 13); anamnestic risk factors, such as obesity and oral contraceptives; or, in cases of major surgical procedures (lasting more than 60 minutes), such as aneurism clipping, exclusion of arteriovenous malformation, exeresis of cavernous malformations, or evacuation of an intracerebral hemorrhage. These patients started a pharmacological prophylaxis with LMWH 5-7 days before surgery, discontinued it the day before the scheduled operation, and restarted it in the second postoperative day to continue the treatment until complete mobilization was achieved (on average 4 days).

Finally, patients were considered at high risk for postoperative DVT in cases of a previous episode of DVT and/or PE, brain or spinal tumors (including benign tumors and malignancies), and concomitant chemo- or radiotherapy. High-risk patients started the pharmacological prophylaxis with LMWH 5-7 days before surgery, discontinued it the day before the scheduled operation and restarted it in the second postoperative day to continue the treatment for 2-3 weeks after their complete mobilization.

Despite the degree of risk, all patients had pre- and postoperative elastic stockings (starting from the day of hospitalization until they were completely mobile) and a perioperative graduate pneumatic sequential leg (thigh or calf) compression device. In the high-risk patients, this mechanical tool was postoperatively kept in place for a minimum of 48 hours or until the beginning of mobilization.

In cases of neurological deterioration, any bleeding in the surgical site was promptly ruled out by a head or spinal CT scan. Furthermore, in cases when there was a clinical suspicion for DVT or PE, a duplex ultrasonography and a chest x-ray plus a perfusion CT scan were respectively performed.

To investigate the relative risk of postoperative bleeding associated with preoperative anticoagulation, 70 patients from our cohort undergoing cranial surgical procedures were randomly selected and stratified according to tumor or non-tumor cases.

Hence, the occurrence of postoperative bleeding was compared among patients either receiving or not receiving preoperative anticoagulation therapy (χ2 test, 95% CI).

Results

The low-risk group accounted for 1,470 patients (38.5%), whereas moderate-risk and high-risk groups accounted for 1,459 (38.2%) and 889 (23.3%) respectively. All patients were entered in a consecutive manner; their detailed data is presented in Table I. Pregnant women with benign brain tumors were excluded from the study because of possible problems with the fetus. Children were also excluded from the present study.

Our prophylactic protocol was well tolerated in all patients. Clinical evidence of DVT occurred in 0.4% of our cohort; one patient died of fatal PE 2 months after surgery. Less than 1% of our patients presented significant postoperative haemorrhaging, mostly after major cranial surgery. If we consider, instead, the clinical outcome, we did not observe any permanent neurological complications from the postoperative bleeding complications and re-operation.

It is well known that prolonged use of heparin can cause a clotting problem. Therefore, we performed a clotting test (the day before and 2 to 3 days after the operation) on all patients, and no blood abnormalities were detected, including in those patients who experienced postoperative hemorrhaging. The platelet count was found to be completely normal as well. The presence of a postoperative hematoma requiring emergency evacuation occurred in 0.4% cases, and in none of those cases did the operating surgeon notice an increased difficulty in achieving a good hemostasis.

A statistical analysis of the data revealed that patients receiving or not receiving preoperative anticoagulants did not disclose any relationship between preoperative anticoagulation therapy and postoperative hematomas because the difference was statistically insignificant (χ^2 test, p = 0.21; 95% CI, 0.73-2.84). Patients' age and sex (χ^2 test) did not differ significantly in the patients with or without postoperative bleeding complications and, therefore, were not considered associated risk factors (multivariate discriminant analysis). [58]

Finally, it has to be noticed that this was not meant as a randomized study; we have not performed a postoperative CT scan on all cranial cases or an MRI on spinal ones, and we have not systematically performed a study to detect any asymptomatic DVT. We have only studied patients who have shown signs or symptoms typical for intracranial bleedings and/or for DVT. Therefore, it is likely that some patients with asymptomatic intracranial bleeding or with DVT have been missed in the analyses.

Table 1. Demographic data of the overall population (presented as percentage)

Baseline characteristics	
Mean age (y)	63.3
Female (%)	54.7
Male (%)	45.3
Cranial cases (n=1375)	
Brain aneurysm (%)	3.6
Arteriovenous malformations (%)	0.9
Cavernous hemangiomas (%)	1.2
Meningioma (%)	5.7
Low-grade glioma (%)	2.2
Central neurocytoma (%)	0.2
High-grade glioma (%)	7.9
Metastasis (%)	8.9
Treumatic intracerebral hemorrhage (%)	4.3
Traumatic extradural hematoma (%)	3.6
Traumatic subdural hematoma (%)	6.3
Spontaneous hypertensive intracerebral hemorrhage (%)	4.5
Decompressive craniectomies with duroplasty (%)	6.4
Stereotactic and /or frameless biopsy (%)	6.0
Chronic subdural hematoma (%)	8.0
Venticuloperitoneal shunts (%)	6.0
External or endoscopic venticulostomy (%)	6.0
Burr hole for open biopsy, cystic tumor drainage (%)	7.5
Miscellaneous cranial procedures (%)	12.8
Spinal cases (n=2443)	
Cervical disk herniation (%)	7.3
Dorsal disk herniation (%)	0.8
Lumber disk herniation (%)	18.7
Multilevel cervical stenosis (%)	12.8
Multilevel lumber stenosis (including spondilolysthesis) (%)	24.4
Cervical fractures (%)	7.0
Dorsal fractures (%)	5.6
Lumbar fractures (%)	5.8
Primary extradural tumors (%)	1.8
Primary intramedullary tumors (%)	1.2
Spinal metastasis (%)	4.7
Vertebroplasty (%)	1.4
Cyphoplasty (%)	3.3
Miscellaneous spinal procedures (%)	4.9

Conclusion

The majority of DVT seems to develop within the first week after a neurosurgical procedure, and a linear correlation between the duration of surgery and DVT occurrence has been highlighted (Khaldhi et al.). The incidence of DVT seems greater for cranial (7.7%) than spinal procedures (1.5%). Although intermittent pneumatic compression devices provided an adequate reduction of DVT/PE in some cranial and combined cranial/spinal series, low-dose subcutaneous UFH or LMWH further reduced the incidence, not always of DVT, but of PE. Nevertheless, low-dose heparin-based prophylaxis in cranial and spinal series risks minor and major postoperative hemorrhages: 2% to 4% in a cranial series, 3.4% minor and 3.4% major hemorrhages in combined cranial/spinal series, and a 0.7% incidence of major/minor hemorrhages in spinal series.

To this regard, contributions to the neurosurgical literature continue to shape, but have yet to clearly define, the appropriate chemoprophylactic use of UFH and LMWH in neurosurgical patients. Ray et al. presented the emerging notionthat DVT is a preventable complication in hospitalized patients that should be approached with caution, and that prospective studies are needed to further elucidate appropriate treatment protocols in both the identification of and the prophylaxis for DVT in neurosurgical patients.

Indeed, the results reported in literature confirm the need for a DVT prophylactic protocol in neurosurgical patients. Nonetheless, there still lacks a prospective randomized trial to assess the best dosage, molecule and timing of LMWH administration. On the other hand, even if our database is limited because of the observational design, the results obtained during the 6 years associated with the application of the DVT prophylactic protocol herein described are striking encouraging. In our institution, the abovementioned protocol clearly showed its efficacy in terms of DVT and PE prevention, and resized the concerns for postoperative complications such as surgical site haemorrhaging.

The wide variability in clinical practice for thromboprophylaxis in neurosurgical patients, in part, is due to the paucity of data based on clinical trials; therefore, further studies, especially randomized ones, are needed to investigate and clarify the best regimen efficacy and the ideal starting and stopping time in terms of safety and efficacy. Without clear guidelines that can be universally applied to this diverse group of patients, prophylaxis for DVT and PE should be tailored to the individual patient with a cautious assessment of benefits versus risks.

References

[1]   Iorio A, Agnelli G. Low-molecular-weight and unfractionated heparin for prevention of venous thromboembolism in neurosurgery: a metanalysis. *Arch. Intern. Med.* 2000; 160: 2327-32.

[2]   Haines ST. Venous thromboembolism: pathophysiology and clinical presentation. *Am. J. Health Syst. Pharm.* 2003; 60 (22 Suppl 7): S3- S5.

[3]   Gallus AS, Salzman EW, Hirsh J. Prevention of venous thromboembolism. In: Colman RW, Hirsh J, Marder, VJ Salzman EW, eds. Hemostasis and Thrombosis: basic principles and clinical practice. 3rd edition Philadelphia. *JB Lippincott* 1994; 1331-45.

[4]   Skillman JJ, Collins RE, Coe NP, Goldstein BS, Shapiro RM, Zervas NT, Bettmann MA, Salzman EW. Prevention of deep vein thrombosis in neurosurgical patients: a controlled, randomized trial of external pneumatic compression boots. *Surgery.* 1978; 83(3): 354-8.

[5]   Cerrato D, Ariano C, Fiacchino F. Deep vein thrombosis and low-dose heparin prophylaxis in neurosurgical patients. *J. Neurosurg.* 1978; 49(3): 378-81.

[6]   Valladares JB, Hankinson J. Incidence of lower extremity deep vein thrombosis in neurosurgical patients. *Neurosurgery.* 1980; 6(2): 138-41.

[7]   Powers SK, Edwards MS. Prophylaxis of thromboembolism in the neurosurgical patient: a review. *Neurosurgery.* 1982; 10(4): 509-13.

[8]   Ruff RL, Posner JB. Incidence and treatment of peripheral venous thrombosis in patients with glioma. *Ann. Neurol.* 1983; 13(3):334-6.

[9]   Boström S, Holmgren E, Jonsson O, Lindberg S, Lindström B, Winsö I, Zachrisson B. Post-operative thromboembolism in neurosurgery. A study on the prophylactic effect of calf muscle stimulation plus dextran compared to low-dose heparin. *Acta Neurochir.* 1986; 80(3-4): 83-9.

[10]   Black PM, Crowell RM, Abbott WM. External pneumatic calf compression reduces deep venous thrombosis in patients with ruptured intracranial aneurysms. *Neurosurgery.* 1986; 18(1): 25-8.

[11]   Black PM, Baker MF, Snook CP. Experience with external pneumatic calf compression in neurology and neurosurgery. *Neurosurgery.* 1986; 18(4): 440-4.

[12]   Bynke O, Hillman J, Lassvik C. Does peroperative external pneumatic leg muscle compression prevent post-operative venous thrombosis in neurosurgery? *Acta Neurochir.* 1987; 88(1-2): 46-8.

[13]   Becker DM, Gonzalez M, Gentili A, Eismont F, Green BA. Prevention of deep venous thrombosis in patients with acute spinal cord injuries: use of rotating treatment tables. *Neurosurgery.* 1987; 20(5): 675-7.

[14]   Turpie AG, Hirsh J, Gent M, Julian D, Johnson J. Prevention of deep vein thrombosis in potential neurosurgical patients. A randomized trial comparing graduated compression stockings alone or graduated compression stockings plus intermittent pneumatic compression with control. *Arch. Intern. Med.* 1989; 149(3): 679-81.

[15]   Bucci MN, Papadopoulos SM, Chen JC, Campbell JA, Hoff JT. Mechanical prophylaxis of venous thrombosis in patients undergoing craniotomy: a randomized trial. *Surg. Neurol.* 1989; 32(4): 285-8.

[16]   Muchmore JH, Dunlap JN, Culicchia F, Kerstein MD. Deep vein thrombophlebitis and pulmonary embolism in patients with malignant gliomas. *South Med. J.* 1989; 82(11): 1352-6.

[17]   Constantini S, Kornowski R, Pomeranz S, Rappaport ZH. Thromboembolic phenomena in neurosurgical patients operated upon for primary and metastatic brain tumors. *Acta Neurochir.* 1991; 109(3-4): 93-7.

[18]   Frim DM, Barker FG 2nd, Poletti CE, Hamilton AJ. Postoperative low-dose heparin decreases thromboembolic complications in neurosurgical patients. *Neurosurgery.* 1992; 30(6): 830-2; discussion 832-3.

[19]   Ferree BA, Wright AM. Deep venous thrombosis following posterior lumbar spinal surgery. *Spine.* 1993; 18(8): 1079-82.

[20]   Ferree BA. Deep venous thrombosis following lumbar laminotomy and laminectomy. *Orthopedics.* 1994; 17(1): 35-8.

[21]   Hamilton MG, Hull RD, Pineo GF. Venous thromboembolism in neurosurgery and neurology patients: a review. *Neurosurgery.* 1994; 34(2): 280-96.

[22]   Wilson JT, Rogers FB, Wald SL, Shackford SR, Ricci MA. Prophylactic vena cava filter insertion in patients with traumatic spinal cord injury: preliminary results. *Neurosurgery.* 1994; 35(2): 234-9.

[23]   Stephens PH, Healy MT, Smith M, Jewkes DA. Prophylaxis against thromboembolism in neurosurgical patients: a survey of current practice in the United Kingdom. *Br. J. Neurosurg.* 1995; 9(2): 159-63.

[24]   Nurmohamed MT, van Riel AM, Henkens CM, Koopman MM, Que GT, d'Azemar P, Büller HR, ten Cate JW, Hoek JA, van der Meer J, van der

Heul C, Turpie AG, Haley S, Sicurella A, Gent M. Low molecular weight heparin and compression stockings in the prevention of venous thromboembolism in neurosurgery. *Thromb. Haemost.* 1996; 75(2): 233-8.

[25] Flinn WR, Sandager GP, Silva MB Jr, Benjamin ME, Cerullo LJ, Taylor M. Prospective surveillance for perioperative venous thrombosis. Experience in 2643 patients. *Arch. Surg.* 1996; 131(5): 472-80.

[26] Agnelli G, Piovella F, Buoncristiani P, Severi P, Pini M, D'Angelo A, Beltrametti C, Damiani M, Andrioli GC, Pugliese R, Iorio A, Brambilla G. Enoxaparin plus compression stockings compared with compression stockings alone in the prevention of venous thromboembolism after elective neurosurgery. *N. Engl. J. Med.* 1998; 339(2): 80-5.

[27] Dickinson LD, Miller LD, Patel CP, Gupta SK. Enoxaparin increases the incidence of postoperative intracranial hemorrhage when initiated preoperatively for deep venous thrombosis prophylaxis in patients with brain tumors. *Neurosurgery.* 1998; 43(5):1074-81.

[28] Wen DY, Hall WA. Complications of subcutaneous low-dose heparin therapy in neurosurgical patients. *Surg. Neurol.* 1998; 50(6): 521-5.

[29] Chan AT, Atiemo A, Diran LK, Licholai GP, McLaren Black P, Creager MA, Goldhaber SZ. Venous thromboembolism occurs frequently in patients undergoing brain tumor surgery despite prophylaxis. *J. Thromb. Thrombolysis.* 1999; 8(2): 139-42.

[30] Macdonald RL, Amidei C, Lin G, Munshi I, Baron J, Weir BK, Brown F, Erickson RK, Hekmatpanah J. Safety of perioperative subcutaneous heparin for prophylaxis of venous thromboembolism in patients undergoing craniotomy. *Neurosurgery.* 1999; 45(2): 245-51; discussion 251-2.

[31] Rossi R, Agnelli G, Taborelli P, Fioroni C, Zerbi D, Pattacini P, Giugni E, Bagatella P, Vaccarino A. Local versus central assessment of venographies in a multicenter trial on the prevention of deep vein thrombosis in neurosurgery. *Thromb. Haemost.* 1999; 82(5): 1399-402.

[32] Agnelli G. Prevention of venous thromboembolism after neurosurgery. *Thromb. Haemost.* 1999; 82(2): 925-30.

[33] Nurmohamed MT. Thromboprophylaxis in neurosurgical patients. *Semin. Hematol.* 2000; 37(3 Suppl 5): 15-8.

[34] Cupitt JM. Prophylaxis against thromboembolism in patients with traumatic brain injury: a survey of UK practice. *Anaesthesia* 2001; 56(8): 780-85.

[35] Wong KC, Boet R, Poon WS, Yu S. Inferior vena caval filters following deep vein thrombosis in patients with ruptured intracranial aneurysm. *Hong Kong Med. J.* 2002; 8(4): 288-90.

[36] Kumar K, Tang KK, Thomas J, Chumpon C. Is postoperative deep vein thrombosis a problem in neurosurgical patients with brain tumours in Singapore? *Singapore Med. J.* 2002; 43(7): 345-9.

[37] Goldhaber SZ, Dunn K, Gerhard-Herman M, Park JK, Black PM. Low rate of venous thromboembolism after craniotomy for brain tumor using multimodality prophylaxis. *Chest.* 2002; 122(6): 1933-7.

[38] Carman TL, Kanner AA, Barnett GH, Deitcher SR. Prevention of thromboembolism after neurosurgery for brain and spinal tumors. *South Med. J.* 2003; 96(1): 17-22.

[39] McDonald RL, Amidei C, Baron J, Weir B, Brown F, Erickson RK, Hekmatpanah J, Frim D. Randomized, pilot study of intermittent pneumatic compression devices plus dalteparin versus intermittent pneumatic compression devices plus heparin for prevention of venous thromboembolism in patients undergoing craniotomy. *Surg. Neurol.* 2003; 59(5): 363-72.

[40] Auguste KI, Quinones-Hinojosa A, Gadkary C, Zada G, Lamborn KR, Berger MS. Incidence of venous thromboembolism in patients undergoing craniotomy and motor mapping for glioma without intraoperative mechanical prophylaxis to the contralateral leg. *J. Neurosurg.* 2003; 99(4): 680-4.

[41] Gerlach R, Scheuer T, Beck J, Woszczyk A, Seifert V, Raabe A. Risk of postoperative hemorrhage after intracranial surgery after early nadroparin administration: results of a prospective study. *Neurosurgery.* 2003; 53(5): 1028-34; discussion 1034-5.

[42] Brambilla S, Ruosi C, La Maida GA, Caserta S. Prevention of venous thromboembolism in spinal surgery. *Eur. Spine. J.* 2004; 13(1): 1-8.

[43] Gerlach R, Raabe A, Beck J, Woszczyk A, Seifert V. Postoperative nadroparin administration for prophylaxis of thromboembolic events is not associated with an increased risk of hemorrhage after spinal surgery. *Eur. Spine. J.* 2004; 13(1): 9-13.

[44] Begelman SM, Green D. Patients undergoing surgical resection of primary brain tumors should receive pharmacologic venous thromboprophylaxis. *Med. Clin. North Am.* 2003; 87(6): 1179-87.

[45] Tabori U, Beni-Adani L, Dvir R, Burstein Y, Feldman Z, Pessach I, Rechavi G, Constantini S, Toren A Risk of venous thromboembolism in

pediatric patients with brain tumors. *Pediatr. Blood Cancer.* 2004; 43(6): 633-6.

[46] Browd SR, Ragel BT, Davis GE, Scott AM, Skalabrin EJ, Couldwell WT. Prophylaxis for deep venous thrombosis in neurosurgery: a review of the literature. *Neurosurg. Focus.* 2004; 17(4): E1.

[47] Danish SF, Burnett MG, Stein SC. Prophylaxis for deep venous thrombosis in patients with craniotomies: a review. *Neurosurg. Focus.* 2004; 17(4): E2.

[48] Smith SF, Simpson JM, Sekhon LH. Prophylaxis for deep venous thrombosis in neurosurgical oncology: review of 2779 admissions over a 9-year period. *Neurosurg. Focus.* 2004; 17(4): E4.

[49] Danish SF, Burnett MG, Ong JG, Sonnad SS, Maloney-Wilensky E, Stein SC. Prophylaxis for deep venous thrombosis in craniotomy patients: a decision analysis. *Neurosurgery.* 2005; 56(6): 1286-92.

[50] Payen JF, Faillot T, Audibert G, Vergnes MC, Bosson JL, Lestienne B, Bernard C, Bruder N. Thromboprophylaxis in neurosurgery and head trauma. *Ann. Fr. Anesth. Reanim.* 2005; 24(8): 921-7.

[51] Audibert G, Faillot T, Vergnes MC, Bosson JL, Bernard C, Payen JF, Lestienne B, Bruder N. Thromboprophylaxis in elective spinal surgery and spinal cord injury. *Ann. Fr. Anesth. Reanim.* 2005; 24(8): 928-34.

[52] Epstein NE. A review of the risks and benefits of differing prophylaxis regimens for the treatment of deep venous thrombosis and pulmonary embolism in neurosurgery. *Surg. Neurol.* 2005; 64(4): 295-301.

[53] Epstein NE. Intermittent pneumatic compression stocking prophylaxis against deep venous thrombosis in anterior cervical spinal surgery: a prospective efficacy study in 200 patients and literature review. *Spine* .2005; 30(22): 2538-43.

[54] Epstein NE. Efficacy of pneumatic compression stocking prophylaxis in the prevention of deep venous thrombosis and pulmonary embolism following 139 lumbar laminectomies with instrumented fusions. *J. Spinal. Disord. Tech.* 2006; 19(1): 28-31.

[55] Smith SF, Biggs MT, Sekhon LH. Risk factors and prophylaxis for deep venous thrombosis in neurosurgery. *Surg. Technol. Int.* 2005; 14: 69-76.

[56] Semrad TJ, O'Donnell R, Wun T, Chew H, Harvey D, Zhou H, White RH. Epidemiology of venous thromboembolism in 9489 patients with malignant glioma. *J. Neurosurg.* 2007; 106(4): 601-8.

[57]   Pechlivanis I, Engelhardt M, Scholz M, Harders A, Schmieder K. Deep venous thrombosis after lumbar disc surgery due to compression of the vena cava caused by a retroperitoneal haematoma. *Eur. Spine. J.* 2008; 17 Suppl 2: S324-6.

[58]   Chibbaro S, Tacconi L. Safety of deep venous thrombosis prophylaxis with low-molecular-weight heparin in brain surgery. Prospective study on 746 patients. *Surg. Neurol.* 2008; 70(2): 117-21.

[59]   Tolani KA, Bendo AA. Prevention and treatment of homeostatic disorders after central neurosurgical procedures. *Best. Pract. Res. Clin. Anaesthesiol.* 2007; 21(4): 539-56.

[60]   Tetri S, Hakala J, Juvela S, Saloheimo P, Pyhtinen J, Rusanen H, Savolainen ER, Hillbom M. Safety of low-dose subcutaneous enoxaparin for the prevention of venous thromboembolism after primary intracerebral haemorrhage. *Thromb. Res.* 2008; 123(2): 206-12.

[61]   Collen JF, Jackson JL, Shorr AF, Moores LK. Prevention of venous thromboembolism in neurosurgery: a metanalysis. *Chest.* 2008; 134(2): 237-49.

[62]   Glotzbecker MP, Bono CM, Harris MB, Brick G, Heary RF, Wood KB. Surgeon practices regarding postoperative thromboembolic prophylaxis after high-risk spinal surgery. *Spine.* 2008; 33(26): 2915-21.

[63]   Glotzbecker MP, Bono CM, Wood KB, Harris MB. Thromboembolic disease in spinal surgery: a systematic review. *Spine.* 2009; 34(3): 291-303.

[64]   Ploumis A, Ponnappan RK, Bessey JT, Patel R, Vaccaro AR. Thromboprophylaxis in spinal trauma surgery: consensus among spine trauma surgeons. *Spine. J.* 2009; 9(7): 530-6.

[65]   Cage TA, Lamborn KR, Ware ML, Frankfurt A, Chakalian L, Berger MS, McDermott MW. Adjuvant enoxaparin therapy may decrease the incidence of postoperative thrombotic events though does not increase the incidence of postoperative intracranial hemorrhage in patients with meningiomas. *J. Neurooncol.* 2009; 93(1): 151-6.

[66]   Nicol M, Sun Y, Craig N, Wardlaw D. Incidence of thromboembolic complications in lumbar spinal surgery in 1,111 patients. *Eur. Spine. J.* 2009; 18(10): 1548-52.

[67]   Niemi T, Silvasti-Lundell M, Armstrong E, Hernesniemi J. The Janus face of thromboprophylaxis in patients with high risk for both thrombosis and bleeding during intracranial surgery: report of five exemplary cases. *Acta. Neurochir.* 2009; 151(10): 1289-94.

[68] Bauman JA, Church E, Halpern CH, Danish SF, Zaghloul KA, Jaggi JL, Stein SC, Baltuch GH. Subcutaneous heparin for prophylaxis of venous thromboembolism in deep brain stimulation surgery: evidence from a decision analysis. *Neurosurgery.* 2009; 65(2): 276-80.

[69] Raslan AM, Fields JD, Bhardwaj A. Prophylaxis for venous thromboembolism in neurocritical care: a critical appraisal. *Neurocrit. Care.* 2010; 12(2): 297-309.

[70] Ploumis A, Ponnappan RK, Sarbello J, Dvorak M, Fehlings MG, Baron E, Anand N, Okonkwo DO, Patel A, Vaccaro AR. Thromboprophylaxis in traumatic and elective spinal surgery: analysis of questionnaire response and current practice of spine trauma surgeons. *Spine* 2010; 35(3): 323-9.

[71] Taniguchi S, Fukuda I, Daitoku K, Minakawa M, Odagiri S, Suzuki Y, Fukui K, Asano K, Ohkuma H. Prevalence of venous thromboembolism in neurosurgical patients. *Heart. Vessels.* 2009; 24(6): 425-8.

[72] Niemi T, Armstrong E. Thromboprophylactic management in the neurosurgical patient with high risk for both thrombosis and intracranial bleeding. *Curr. Opin. Anaesthesiol.* 2010; 23(5): 558-63.

[73] Khaldi A, Helo N, Schneck MJ, Origitano TC. Venous thromboembolism: deep venous thrombosis and pulmonary embolism in a neurosurgical population. *J. Neurosurg.* 2011; 114(1): 40-6.

[74] Michiels JJ, Gadisseur A, Van Der Planken M, Schroyens W, De Maeseneer M, Hermsen JT, Trienekens PH, Hoogsteden H, Pattynama PM. A critical appraisal of non-invasive diagnosis and exclusion of deep vein thrombosis and pulmonary embolism in outpatients with suspected deep vein thrombosis or pulmonary embolism: how many tests do we need? *Int. Angiol.* 2005; 24(1): 27-39.

[75] Roderick P, Ferris G, Wilson K, Halls H, Jackson D, Collins R, Baigent C. Towards evidence-based guidelines for the prevention of venous thromboembolism: systematic reviews of mechanical methods, oral anticoagulation, dextran and regional anaesthesia as thromboprophylaxis. *Health Technology Assessment.* 2005; 9(49): 1-91.

[76] Hak DJ. Prevention of venous thromboembolism in trauma and long bone fractures. *Curr. Opin. Pulm. Med.* 2001; 7(5): 338-43.

[77] Britt LD, Zolfaghari D, Kennedy E, Pagel KJ, Minghini A. Incidence and prophylaxis of deep vein thrombosis in a high risk trauma population. *Am. J. Surg.* 1996; 172(1): 13-4.

[78] Streiff MB. Vena cava filters: a review for intensive care specialists. *J. Intensive Care Med.* 2003; 18(2): 59-79.

[79] Hirsh J, Dalen JE, Guyatt G. The sixth ACCP guidelines on antithrombotic therapy for prevention and treatment of thrombosis. *Chest.* 2001; 119; 1S-2S.

In: Deep Vein Thrombosis
Editor: Takashi Yamaki

ISBN: 978-1-62257-519-0
© 2013 Nova Science Publishers, Inc.

Chapter 4

Combination of Pretest Clinical Probability Score and Different D-dimer Cutoff Value for Exclusion of Venous Thromboembolism

*Takashi Yamaki**
Department of Plastic and Reconstructive Surgery,
Tokyo Women's Medical University, Shinjuku-ku, Tokyo, Japan

Abstract

Prompt diagnosis of venous deep vein thromboembolism (VTE) is mandatory, but only 25% of suspected cases are confirmed by objective testing. In this background, the D-dimer testing with high negative predictive value represents an excellent triage test in patients with suspected VTE. In general, enzyme-liked immunosorbent assay (ELISA) offers the best of current D-dimer assay for sensitivity. Latex quantitative assay and whole-blood assay might also represent valid alternative for

* Correspondence to: Professor Takashi Yamaki MD, Department of Plastic and Reconstructive Surgery, Tokyo Women's Medical University, 8-1, Kawada-cho, Shinjuku-ku, Tokyo, 162-8666, Japan. Tel: +81-3-3353-8111. Fax: +81-3-3225-0940.
E-mail: yamaki@prs.twmu.ac.jp, Yamakit@aol.com.

exclusion of VTE. Recently, a combination of pretest clinical probability (PTP) score and D-dimer testing has been considered validated as a diagnostic strategy for pulmonary embolism or deep vein thrombosis (DVT). This strategy is specifically validated for patients who have low PTP. Even the combination of low PTP and a normal D-dimer concentration can be considered a safe strategy to withhold anticoagulation in patients with suspected VTE.

D-dimer cutoff value also affects the discriminating power. The sensitivity could be improved by lowering the cutoff value, but the subsequent decrease in specificity would lead to a large number of false-positive results. On the contrary, D-dimer assays with very high specificity provide fewer false-positive results, but they are less sensitive for VTE and cannot be used to exclude the disease in all patients. In this background, we analyzed if varying the D-dimer cutoff according to PTP would exclude VTE in more patients than using the single D-dimer cutoff point. Using latex agglutination assay, we found that D-dimer cutoff points of 2.6, 1.1 and 1.1µg/mL were selected for the low, moderate and high PTP groups among 886 patients with suspected DVT. In the low PTP group, specificity increased from 48.9% to 78.2% (P <0.0001) with use of the different D-dimer cutoff value. In the moderate and high risk PTP groups, however, the different D-dimer levels did not achieve substantial improvement. Regardless, overall venous duplex scanning could have been reduced by 43.0% using different D-dimer cutoff points. Even in patients with proven PE, a combination of a specific D-dimer level and PTP score is most effective in the low PTP patients in excluding DVT.

In summary, a combination of PTP score and different D-dimer cutoff provides an effective means in terms of avoiding a large number of unnecessary venous duplex scanning in suspected symptomatic DVT in the low PTP for DVT.

Introduction

Venous thromboembolism (VTE) is a common disorder with morbidity and potential for mortality. Currently, more than 600,000 cases of pulmonary embolism (PE) occur with an estimated annual incidence of 23-69 per 100,000 population in the United States alone [1-3]. Since PE is potentially life-threatening, and 80% of cases arise from lower extremity veins [4], diagnosis and treatment of deep vein thrombosis (DVT) is of primary importance. However, accurate diagnosis of venous thromboembolism (VTE) still remains a difficult challenge for clinicians. Clinical signs and symptoms are inaccurate, and so that an accurate diagnostic test is mandatory to exclude VTE. Diagnostic imaging using contrast venography or venous duplex ultrasound has several limitations. Venography is invasive and expensive, is contraindicated in patients who are allergic to contrast media. Venous duplex scan has high sensitivity for diagnosis of proximal DVT and has been becoming as a gold standard for DVT, but it has poor sensitivity for detection of calf vein thrombosis. If the initial scan is proven to be negative, serial testing is often required which is also disadvantage to be expensive and time-consuming. The pretest clinical probability (PTP) score developed by Wells et al. [5] is useful triage tool to select patients who have to be further evaluated for DVT by imaging tests. The PTP score uses explicit medical history and physical examination criteria to stratify patients into low, moderate, and high risk of DVT. Another useful triage tool to decrease the unnecessary imaging tests is D-dimer assay. Using a D-dimer test with a high negative predictive value (NPV), presence of DVT is safely excluded [6]. In recent years, several authors have evaluated the role of D-dimer assay as an adjunct to the pretest clinical probability score. Therefore, this Chapter presents the feasibility of clinical strategy for excluding DVT on the basis of a combination of D-dimer testing and PTP score.

Pretest Clinical Probability Score

In the past, many patients presumed to have VTE on the basis of clinical signs and symptoms alone had been incorrectly diagnosed and inappropriately.

Table 1. Pretest Clinical Probability Score for DVT

Active cancer (treatment ongoing) or within previous 6 months or palliative	+1
Paralysis, paresis, or recent plaster immobilization of the lower extremity	+1
Recently bedridden for more than 3 days or major surgery within 4 weeks	+1
Localized tenderness along the distribution of the deep venous system	+1
Entire leg swollen	+1
Calf swelling by > 3cm when compared with the asymptomatic leg (measured below tibial tuberosity)	+1
Pitting edema	+1
Collateral superficial veins (nonvaricose)	+1
Alternative diagnosis as likely as or more likely than DVT	+1
Low risk (≤ 0 points)	
Moderate risk (1-2 points)	
High risk (3 ≥ points)	

The clinical diagnosis of VTE is often unreliable without objective testing. While studies have shown that individual signs and symptoms in patients with suspected VTE are mostly unreliable [7, 8], the clinical assessment has re-emerged as an adjunctive tool for exclusion of VTE with appropriate diagnostic examinations.

The clinical models to predict PTP of DVT have been developed and evaluated for the usefulness to exclude the diagnosis of DVT, which can effectively stratify patients with suspected DVT into low-, moderate-, or high probability groups (Table 1).

Using this crireria, Wells and associates found that patients in the high risk PTP group had a 75% chance of DVT compared with 17% and 3% chance in the moderate and low risk groups, respectively. They found that the difference in prevalence of DVT in the three categories was statistically significant, and concluded that combination of patients' PTP with venous duplex ultrasound results had the potential to simplify and improve the diagnostic process in patients with suspected DVT [9]. This strategy has become the most widely accepted prediction rule for DVT. Several studies have also investigated the PTP assessment in patients with PE in both inpatients and outpatients [10-12]. However, the variability of the sensitivity and NPV between the different risk categories limits the usefulness of PTP as a single exclusionary selection test.

D-dimer Assay

The D-dimer is a specific fragment produced during the degradation of fibrin, and the D-dimer assay is a promising adjunctive tool for non-invasive diagnostic management of patients with suspected DVT. Several methods are commercially available for measuring D-dimer concentrations: (1) latex agglutination, (2) microplate ELISA, (3) immunofiltration (membrane ELISA), and (4) whole-blood agglutination.

Among various D-dimer tests, ELISA-based techniques have the highest sensitivity and NPV for DVT, and are considered to be the gold standard in determining D-dimer [13-19]. But they are time-consuming and not suitable for emergency use.

The first-generation latex agglutination assays are based on the visible agglutination of antibody-coated latex particles. Positive samples may be serially diluted to provide a semi-quantitative estimate of the D-dimer concentration. Although these assays are rapid and easy to perform, the results are qualitative, observer-dependent, and limited in their ability to detect minimally increased D-dimer concentrations. The second-generation latex immunoassays employ the same basic technique as the first-generation assays, but use a photometric analyzer to provide a quantitative measure of the D-dimer and are generally able to measure lower concentrations of D-dimer reproducibly [20]. Among 556 consecutive outpatients with a suspected first episode of DVT, Bates et al. demonstrated a NPV of 99.7% (CI, 98.2% to 100%), a sensitivity of 98.2% (CI, 90.4% to 100%), and a specificity of 60.4% (CI, 56.1% to 64.7%) for exclusion of DVT using an automated, second-generation quantitative latex MDAD-Dimer assay® (Organon Teknika Corp., now bioMérieux, Inc., Durham, North Carolina) [21]. Although the prevalence of DVT was only 10%, they also showed that 50.9% of the patients with a low or moderate pretest probability and a negative D-dimer result could safely be excluded from further testing. Schutgens evaluated four new D-dimer assays and a classical ELISA in symptomatic outpatients with suspected DVT, and concluded that the Tina-quant® latex assay (Roche, Mannheim, Germany) had the highest negative predictive value of 98%, and a high sensitivity of 99%, using a standard cut-off value [22].

Wells et al. evaluated 214 patients with clinically suspected deep vein thrombosis using the SimpliRED D-dimer assay, which had a sensitivity of 93% for proximal deep vein thrombosis and a NPV of 98% [23]. Turkstra et al. also found similar accuracy when using the SimpliRED assay [24]. But other investigators demonstrated that this method has relatively low sensitivity for DVT [25, 26]. Again, D-dimer is a product of fibrin degradation by plasmin, and is generated in the presence of thrombus. The D-dimer testing, therefore, is expected to increase in relation to the extent of the thrombus process. Furthermore, D-dimer assays may be positive in patients with other conditions that could activate the coagulation and fibrinolytic cascade [27-29]. Caution should be exercised when considering the use of this assay as the sole exclusionary pre-selection test for the evaluation of DVT [30].

Combination of PTP and D-dimer Assay for Exclusion of DVT

The use of D-dimer assay with recommended cut-off value combined with PTPs been established as an adjunct to the venous duplex ultrasound by many

[25, 26, 28, 29, 31-33]. Combination of these methods has the ability to make the diagnosis of DVT more convenient and economical. When considering proximal DVT, this combination provided a sensitivity and NPV of 100% [26]. Similarly, this combination had a sensitivity of 82% and NPV of 97% for isolated calf vein thrombosis, which showed no significant decrease compared to proximal DVT [26].

Several investigators propose that patients with a low PTP and a normal D-dimer concentration do not need further vascular investigations [26, 31, 34]. This approach will reduce the need for venous duplex scanning. And the use of D-dimer testing also reduces the need for repeated venous duplex ultrasound without thromboembolic complications in patients who are likely to have DVT and establishes a definitive diagnosis on the day of presentation in a larger proportion of the patients [35]. Anderson et al. showed that observed NPV of D–dimer using SimpliRed assay was 100% in the low probability patients, 94.1% in moderate probability patients, and 86.7% in high probability patients [33].

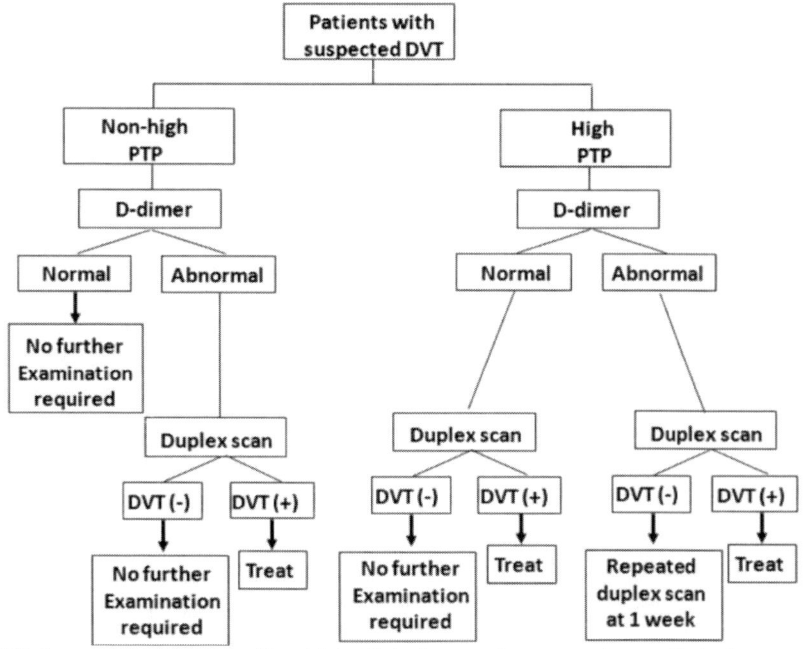

DVT: deep vein thrombosis, Non-high clinical score: low or moderate clinical score. Derived from Yamaki T, et al., *J. Am. Coll. Surg.* 2005; 201: 701-9 [36].

Figure 1. Strategy for patients with suspected DVT.

He concluded that D-dimer assay may be a potentially useful adjunctive test to exclude the diagnosis of DVT in patients at low pretest clinical probability. Furthermore, Schutgens et al. showed that DVT could be also excluded in patients with normal D-dimer concentration and a low and moderate PTP [34]. He used latex agglutination D-dimer assay to fulfill the strategy because the sensitivity of the SimpliRED D-dimer assay was only 85%. As described previously, ELISA D-dimer has the highest sensitivity and NPV for DVT, we found that the excellent sensitivity and NPV of 100% were maintained in each PTP group at a cutoff level of 0.5µg/mL [36]. To exclude DVT, the PTP and the D-dimer testing are recommended instead of using the D-dimer testing alone (Figure 1). For exclusion of DVT in patients with a non-high PTP and a normal D-dimer concentration, we recommend the use of D-dimer assay with the sensitivity and the NPV of nearly 100%.

Combined Use of PTP and Different D-dimer Cutoff Value for Exclusion of DVT

Another factor that could affect the discriminatory power of studies for DVT is the cutoff value of the D-dimer test. The sensitivity could be improved by lowering the cutoff value, but the subsequent decrease in specificity would lead to a large number of false-positive results. On the contrary, D-dimer cutoff values with very high specificity provide fewer false-positive results, but they are less sensitive for DVT and cannot be used to exclude the disease in all patients.

Against this background, two studies concluded that an increased cutoff values of D-dimer reduced the false positives but increased the percentage of false negatives. On the contrary, another study demonstrated that increasing the D-dimer cutoff values led to rise in specificity without loss of sensitivety [37-39]. Using data from a previously published study of 571 patients, Linkins et al. reported that varying the D-dimer cutoff values according to the PTP score would have excluded VTE in more patients than if a single D-dimer cutoff point had been used [40]. In that analysis, they found that in the high PTP score group a D-dimer cutoff point of 0.2 µg FEU mL^{-1} was required to achieve a NPV of 98% or higher. Similarly, in the low PTP score group, a D-dimer cut-off point of 2.1 µg FEU mL^{-1} achieved a NPV of 98% or higher. Using this strategy, the number of patients with false-positive results also dropped from 89 to 9 in the low PTP group (n=205).

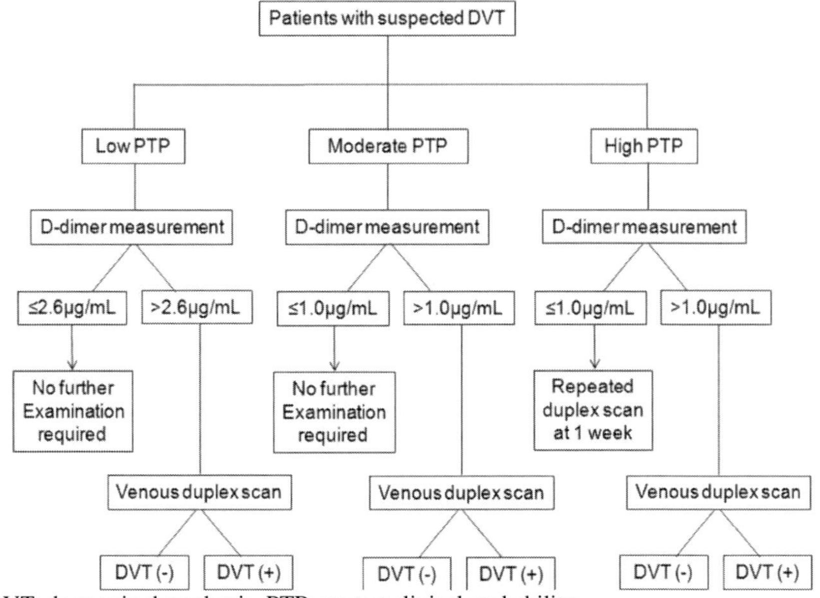

DVT: deep vein thrombosis, PTP: pretest clinical probability.
Derived from Yamaki T, et al., *J. Vasc. Surg.* 2009; 50: 1099-105 [42].

Figure 2. Potential new diagnostic strategy for diagnosis of DVT using different D-dimer levels.

Even in patients with established pulmonary embolism, we demonstrated that combination of a specific D-dimer level for the ELISA D-dimer assay with PTP score is effective for excluding DVT in low-risk PTP patients [41]. We also investigated the utility of a combination of different cutoff points for the latex agglutination D-dimer assay and PTP score to reduce the use of venous duplex scanning in 886 patients with suspected DVT [42]. In that study, 45.9% (233/508) of patients with low PTP scores showed false-positive results when a single cutoff point of 1.0 µg/mL was used. When a specific D-dimer cutoff point of 2.6 µg/mL was selected for low-risk PTP patients, the proportion with false-positive results dropped from 45.9% to 20.5% (104/508), a 25.4% change. Reducing the number of false-positive results could decrease the number of unnecessary venous duplex scans, thus saving both time and money.

These results potentially provided a new strategy for diagnosis of DVT, as demonstrated in Figure 2. Patients who have a low PTP score and a D-dimer level of ≤2.6µg/mL require no further investigation, while patients with a low PTP score and a D-dimer level of >2.6 µg/mL undergo a single venous duplex scan at presentation. Patients who have a moderate PTP score and a normal D-dimer level require no further investigation, and patients who have a moderate PTP score with an elevated D-dimer level should undergo a single venous duplex scan at presentation. Finally, patients with a high PTP score who have an elevated D-dimer level and an initial negative scan undergo a repeat venous duplex scan after one week because they have quite a high risk of DVT.

Conclusion

A combination of a specific D-dimer level with the clinical probability score is an effective approach for excluding DVT in low-risk PTP patients. In patients with moderate or high PTP, however, the recommended cutoff point may be preferable. Results obtained these studies show that the use of different D-dimer levels for patients with different levels of risk is feasible when using different D-dimer assays for excluding DVT.

References

[1]   Anderson FA, Wheeler HB, Goldberg RT, Hosmer DW, Patwardhan NA, Jovanovic B, Forcier A, Dalen JE. A population-based perspective of the hospital incidence and case-fatality rates of deep vein thrombosis and pulmonary embolism: the Worcester DVT Study. *Arch. Intern. Med.* 1991; 151: 933-8.

[2]   Dalen JE, Alpert JS. Natural history of pulmonary embolism. *Prog. Cardiovasc. Dis.* 1975; 17: 259-70.

[3]   Dismuke SE, Wagner EH. Pulmonary embolism as a cause of death. The changing mortality in hospitalized patients. *JAMA.* 1986; 255: 2039-42.

[4]   Sandler DA, Martin JF. Autopsy proven pulmonary embolism in hospital patients: are we detecting enough deep vein thrombosis? *J. R. Soc. Med.* 1989; 82: 203-5.

[5]   Wells PS, Hirsh J, Anderson DR, Lensing AW, Foster G, Kearon C, Weitz JI, D'Ovidio R, Cogo A, Prandoni P, Girolami A, Ginsberg JS. Accuracy of clinical assessment of deep-vein thrombosis. *Lancet.* 1995; 345: 1326-30.

[6]   Stein PD, Hull RD, Patel KC, Olson RE, Ghali WA, Brant R, Biel RK, Bharadia V, Kalra NK. D-dimer for the exclusion of acute venous

thrombosis and pulmonary embolism: a systematic review. *Ann. Intern.Med.* 2004; 140: 589-602.

[7] Anand SS, Wells PS, Hunt D, Brill-Edward P, Cook D, Ginsberg JS. Does this patient have deep vein thrombosis? *JAMA.* 1988; 279: 1094-9.

[8] Kahn SR. The clinical diagnosis of deep venous thrombosis. *Arch. Intern. Med.*1998; 158: 2315-23.

[9] Wells PS, Anderson DR, Bormanis J, Guy F, Mitchell M, Gray L, Clement C, Robinson KS, Lewandowski B. Values of assessment of pretest probability of deep vein thrombosis in clinical management. *Lancet.* 1997; 350: 1795-8.

[10] The PIOPED Investigators. Values of the ventilation/perfusion scan in acute pulmonary embolism. *JAMA.* 1990; 263: 2753-9.

[11] Musset D, Parent F, Meyer G, Maitre S, Girard P, Leroyer C, Revel M, Carette M, Laurent M, Charbonnier B, Laurent F, Mal H, Nonent M, Lancar R, Grenier P, Simonneau G. Diagnostic strategy fr patients with suspected pulmonary embolism: a prospective multi-centre outcome study. *Lancet.* 2002; 360: 1914-20.

[12] Perrier A, Miron M, Desmarais S, de Moerloose P, Slosman D, Didier D, Unger P, Junod A, Patenaude J, Bounameaux H. Using clinical evaluation and lung scan to rule out suspected pulmonary embolism: is it a valid option in patients with normal results of lower-limb venous compression ultrasonography?. *Arch. Intern. Med.* 2000; 160: 512-6.

[13] Elias A, Aptel I, Huc B, Chalé JJ, Nguyen F, Cambus JP, Boccalon H, Boneu B. D-Dimer test and diagnosis of deep vein thrombosis. A comparative study of 7 assays. *Thromb. Haemost.*1996; 76: 518-22.

[14] Freyburger G, Trillaud H, Labrouche S, Gauthier P, Javorschi S, Bernard P, Grenier N. D-Dimer strategy in thrombosis exclusion – a gold standard study in 100 patients suspected of deep venous thrombosis or pulmonary embolism: 8 DD methods compared. *Thromb. Haemost.* 1998; 79: 32-7.

[15] Fünfsinn N, Caliezi C, Biasiutti FD, KorteW, Z'Brun A, Baumgartner I, Ulrich M, Cottier C, Lämmle B, Wuillemin WA. Rapid D-dimer testing and pre-test clinical probability in the exclusion of deep venous thrombosis in symptomatic outpatients. *Blood. Coagul. Fibrinolysis.* 2001; 12: 165-70.

[16] Janssen MC, Heebels AE, de Metz M, Verbruggen H, Wollersheim H, Janssen S, Schuurmans MM, Nová ková IR. Reliability of five rapid D-dimer assays compared to ELISA® in the exclusion of deep venous thrombosis. *Thromb.Haemost.* 1997; 77: 262-6.

[17]   Rowbotham BJ, Carroll P, Whitaker AN, Bunce IH, Cobcroft RG, Elms MJ, Masci PP, Bundesen PG, Rylatt DB, Webber AJ. Measurement of crosslinked fibrin derivatives – use in the diagnosis of venous thrombosis. *Thromb. Haemost.*1987; 57: 59–61.

[18]   van der Graaf F, van den Borne H, van der Kolk M, de Wild PJ, Janssen GW, van Uum SH. Exclusion of deep venous thrombosis with D-dimer testing – comparison of 13 D-dimer methods in 99 outpatients suspected of deep venous thrombosis using venography as reference standard. *Thromb. Haemost.*2000; 83: 191-8.

[19]   Brown MD, Rowe BH, Reeves MJ, Bermingham JM, Goldhaber SZ. The accuracy of the enzyme-linked immunosorbent assay D-dimer test in the diagnosis of pulmonary embolism: a meta-analysis. *Ann. Emerg. Med.* 2002; 40: 133–44.

[20]   Heim SW, Schectman JM, Siadaty MS, Philbrick JT. D-dimer testing for deep venous thrombosis: a metaanalysis. *Clin. Chem.* 2004; 50: 1136-1147.

[21]   Bates SM, Kearon C, Crowther M, Linkins L, O'Donnell M, Douketis J, Lee AYY, Weitz JI, Johnston M, Ginsberg JS. A diagnostic strategy involving a quantitative latex D-dimer assay reliably excludes deep venous thrombosis. *Ann. Intern. Med.* 2003; 138: 783-794.

[22]   Schutgens REG, Haas FJLM, Gerritsen WBM, van der Horst F, Nieuwenhuis HK, Biesma DH. The usefulness of five D-dimer assays in the exclusion of deep vein thrombosis. *J. Thromb. Haemost.* 2003; 1: 976-81.

[23]   Wells PS, Brill-Edwards P, Stevens P, Panju A, Patel A, Douketis J, Massicotte MP, Hirsh J, Weitz JI, Kearon C. A novel and rapid whole-blood assay for D-dimer in patients with clinically suspected deep vein thrombosis. *Circulation.* 1995; 91:2184-7.

[24]   Turkstra F, van Beek EJ, ten Cate JW, Büller HR. Reliable rapid blood test for the exclusion of venous thromboembolism in symptomatic outpatients. *Thromb. Haemost.* 1996; 76:9-11.

[25]   James S, Ashford N. Use of a simplified clinical scoring system and D-dimer testing can reduce the requirement for radiology in the exclusion of deep vein thrombosis by over 20%. *Br. J. Haematol.* 2001; 112: 1079-82.

[26]   Kearon C, Ginsberg JS, Douketis J, Turpie AG, Bates SM, Lee AY, Crowther MA, Weitz JI, Brill-Edwards P, Wells P, Anderson DR, Kovacs MJ, Linkins LA, Julian JA, Bonilla LR, Gent M; Canadian Pulmonary Embolism Diagnosis Study (CANPEDS) Group.

Management of suspected deep vein thrombosis in outpatients by using clinical assessment and D-dimer testing. *Ann. Intern. Med.* 2001; 135: 108-11.

[27] Bounameax H, de Moerloose P, Perrier A, Reber G. Plasma measurement of D-dimer as diagnostic aid in suspected venous thromboembolism: an overview. *Thromb. Haemost.* 1994; 71: 1-6.

[28] Rowbotham B, Whitaker AN, Masci P. D-dimer antibodies. Powerful reagents for the study of human thrombosis and fiblynolysis. *Fibrinolysis.* 1993; 7 (Suppl 2): 9-11.

[29] Anderson DR, Kovacs JM, Kovacs G, Stiell I, Mitchell M, Khoury V, Dryer J, Ward J, Wells PS. Combined use of clinical assessment and D-dimer to improve the management of patients presenting to the emergency department with suspected deep vein thrombosis (the EDITED Study). *J. Thromb. Haemost.* 2003; 1: 645-51.

[30] Brill-Edwards P, Lee A. D-dimer testing in the diagnosis of acute venous thromboembolism. *Thromb. Haemost.* 1999; 82: 688-94.

[31] Lennox AF, Delis KT, Serunkuma S, Zarka ZA, Daskalopoulou SE, Nicolaides AN. Combination of a clinical risk assessment score and rapid whole blood D-dimer testing in the diagnosis of deep vein thrombosis in symptomatic patients. *J. Vasc. Surg.* 1999; 30: 794-804.

[32] Dryjski M, O'Brien-Irr MS, Harris LM, Hassett J, Janicke D. Evaluation of a screen protocol to exclude the diagnosis of deep vein thrombosis among emergency department patients. *J. Vasc. Surg.* 2001; 34: 1010-5.

[33] Anderson DR, Wells PS, Stiell I, MacLeod B, Simms M, Gray L, Robinson KS, Bormanis J, Mitchell M, Lewandowski B, Flowerdew G. Management of patients with suspected deep vein thrombosis in the emergency department: combining use of a clinical diagnosis model with D-dimer testing. *J. Emerg. Med.* 2000; 19: 225-30.

[34] Schutgens REG, Ackermark P, Haas FJLM, Nieuwenhuis HK, Peltenburg HG, Pijlman AH, Pruijm M, Oltmans R, Kelder JC, Biesma DH. Combination of a normal D-dimer concentration and a non-high pretest clinical probability score is a safe strategy to exclude deep venous thrombosis. *Circulation.* 2003; 107: 593-7.

[35] Wells PS, Anderson DR, Rodger M, orgie M, Kearon C, Dreyer J, Kovacs G, Mitchell M, Lewandowski B, Kovacs MJ. Evaluation of D-dimer in the diagnosis of suspected deep vein thrombosis. *N. Engl. J. Med.* 2003; 349: 1227-35.

[36] Yamaki T, Nozaki M, Sakurai H, Takeuchi M, Soejima K, Kono T. Prospective evaluation of a screening protocol to exclude the deep vein

thrombosis on the basis of a combination of quantitative D-dimer testing and pretest clinical probability score. *J. Am. Coll. Surg.* 2005; 201: 701-9.

[37] Harper PL, Theakstone E, Ahmed J, Ockelford P. D-Dimer concentration increases with age reducing the clinical value of the D-Dimer assay in the elderly. *Intern. Med. J.* 2007; 37: 607-613.

[38] Righini M, Goehring C, Bounameaux H, Perrier A. Effect of age on the performance of common diagnostic tests for pulmonary embolism. *Am. J. Med.* 2000; 109: 357-361.

[39] Righini M, de Moerloose P, Reber G, Perrir A, Bounameaux H. Should the D-Dimer cut off value be increased in elderly patients suspected of pulmonary embolism? *Thromb. Haemost.* 2001; 85: 744.

[40] Linkins L-A, Bates SM, Ginsberg JS, Kearon C. Use of different D-dimer level to exclude venous thromboembolism depending on clinical pretest. *J. Thromb. Haemost.* 2004; 2: 1256-60.

[41] Yamaki T, Nozaki M, Sakurai H, Takeuchi M, Kono T, Soejima K. Uses of different D-dimer levels can reduce the need for venous duplex scanning to rule out deep vein thrombosis in patients with symptomatic pulmonary embolism. *J. Vasc. Surg.* 2007; 46: 526-32.

[42] Yamaki T, Nozaki M, Sakurai H, kikuchi Y, Soejima K, Kono T, Hamahata A, Kim K. Combined use of pretest clinical probability score and latex agglutination D-dimer testing for excluding acute deep vein thrombosis. *J. Vasc. Surg.* 2009; 50: 1099-105.

In: Deep Vein Thrombosis
Editor: Takashi Yamaki

ISBN: 978-1-62257-519-0
© 2013 Nova Science Publishers, Inc.

Chapter 5

Ambulatory Treatment of Deep Vein Thrombosis

*Mehmet Kurtoglu**
Department of General Surgery,
Istanbul University, Istanbul School of Medicine,
Capa-Istanbul, Turkey

Abstract

Various options are available for the treatment of deep vein thrombosis (DVT) while the natural course of the disease without intervention results in 30% pulmonary embolus and 10% mortality.

Despite the evident consensus on the high efficacy of anticoagulant and thrombolytic treatments in the prevention of pulmonary embolus in the scientific era, these treatment options are known to be less effective in the prevention of post-thrombotic syndrome (PTS) which is another potential complication. In this respect, thrombolytic treatment has become the main therapeutic option recommended for ilio-femoral DVT which has been considered associated with higher PTS possibility. However, since the past clinical trials on ambulatory conservative anticoagulant treatment were based on the old literature during the former

* Correspondence to: Prof. Dr. Mehmet Kurtoglu, Department of Emergency Surgery, Istanbul University, Istanbul School of Medicine, 34390, Capa-Istanbul, Turkey, Tel: +90-212-236 45 45, Fax: +90-212-236 45 44.
E-mail: metlevkurt@superonline.com.

decade, comparison of this treatment with the recent thrombolytic treatment approach seems to be neither reasonable nor appropriate. Furthermore, there are no randomized clinical trials concerning the direct comparison of thrombolytic and anticoagulant treatments as of yet. Attractive trial results will be published soon but they may also not be able to answer all of the questions.

In this regard, we performed a clinical multi-center study based on an 18-month follow-up of 250 patients in order to evaluate the clinical outcome of neglected ambulatory conservative treatment in detail. According to the results of this study, conservative treatment was determined to be an effective and successful treatment alternative, associated with high total re-canalization ratios reaching 80%, especially in ilio-femoral DVT. When considered in terms of PTS, conservative treatment was also associated with high patient satisfaction with respect to complaints of the patients. For these reasons, we declare conventional conservative treatment to be the most ideal alternative in consensus meeting having level of evidence 1A with comparable and even preferable results in terms of better cost-effectiveness to thrombolytic treatment.

Introduction

Leading to secondary complications like pulmonary thromboembolism, chronic venous insufficiency (post-thrombotic syndrome), chronic pulmonary hypertension and recurrent thrombosis [1, 2]; deep venous thrombosis (DVT) of the lower limbs is a serious disorder associated with significant morbidity and mortality [3, 4].

Having level of evidence 1A, ambulatory treatment has been the treatment used by most physicians for patients with acute DVT [5]. In current practice, the most commonly selected therapeutic options have been documented to be low molecular weight heparin (LMWH) (79.5%), compression stockings (62.3%), unfractionated heparin (UFH; 20.5%), thrombolysis (2.9%) and inferior vena cava (IVC) filter (4.1%), respectively, while one third of patients were identified to be entirely treated out of the hospital [6]. Standard treatments of acute DVT consists of anticoagulation with unfractionated or LMWH followed by oral anticoagulants [7] and past studies have shown that a period of at least 3 months is the optimal duration of oral anticoagulant therapy for proximal DVT [8-11].

Thrombolytic treatment or surgical thrombectomy become therapeutic options in the treatment in selected patient populations provided that serious clinical findings are evident in the legs indicating risk of venous gangrene formation that necessitates urgent removal of the clot. Besides, IVC filters become the therapeutic option in case of bleeding-related complications, a contraindication to the use of anticoagulation and/or failure of the anticoagulation or other options in treating emboli [12].

In this review, the significance of ambulatory treatment of lower limb DVT in comparison to treatment strategies of thrombus removal such as systemic thrombolysis, intrathrombus catheter-directed thrombolysis, contemporary venous thrombectomy and pharmacomechanical thrombolysis is presented with respect to results of the recent national, single arm, prospective, multi-center and open label "THROMBOTEK" trial designed to investigate the long-term (18 months) efficacy and safety of once-daily enoxaparin as a bridge to warfarin for the outpatient ambulatory treatment of lower-limb venous thromboembolism (VTE).

Significance of DVT

DVTs affect around 56-122 individuals per 100,000 in the general population per year. In the USA, DVTs are responsible for 50,000-200,000 deaths annually, at the same time representing the third most common cardiovascular pathology in the UK after coronary artery disease and stroke [13-15].

Up to 30% of hospitalized patients have asymptomatic non-obstructive calf vein thromboses. DVT occurs in more than 20% of patients having major surgery and 40% of those having major orthopedic surgery. A weighted mean incidence of first-time DVT in the general population was documented to be 5.04 per 10,000 person a year [16, 17].

Morbidity of patients with DVT is high even years after the initial event. Besides the risk of acute pulmonary embolism (PE), DVT is associated with a variety of symptoms, generally referred to as "post-thrombotic syndrome" (PTS) [18].

One of the significant complications associated with DVTs, pulmonary emboli become the major debate identified in 30% of untreated cases and leading to 10% of inpatient deaths [14, 17]. Of two million people in the United States who develop DVT, nearly 100,000 sustain fatal pulmonary emboli [19]. VTE is the number one preventable cause of death in hospitalized patients [20]. Approximately 300,000 individuals die of PE every year and deaths from PE are 5 times more common than deaths from breast cancer, motor vehicle accidents, and AIDS combined [12].

Approximately two-thirds of patients with ilio-femoral DVT are known to develop PTS within 1–5 years of the acute thrombosis, symptoms of which preceded by venous valvular incompetence [7]. PTS develops in all untreated cases within 10 years with an increased risk for each year passed without treatment [18]. It is estimated that up to 80% of patients with a DVT may go on to develop symptoms of PTS, while 4-15% progress to leg ulceration [15]. Patients with PTS (pain and leg swelling after thrombosis) suffer poor quality of life due to chronic symptoms. The incidence of PTS is as high as 30% over 8 years [21].

Management of Iliofemoral DVT

Major goals of DVT treatment are to prevent the development of pulmonary emboli which is one of the fatal complications of the disease leading to pulmonary hypertension, to minimize risk of PTS and to prevent the recurrence and optimize resolution of thrombus. Accordingly, restoring venous patency and valve function are surrogate outcomes while incidence of PTS, quality of life and DVT recurrence are of primary importance in the long-term outcome of ilio-femoral DVT [17, 22].

Current therapeutic options in the management of ilio-femoral DVT are ambulatory treatment, thrombolytic treatment, and surgical thrombectomy and if thrombolytic treatment or surgical thrombectomy is not possible or is contraindicated, IVC filters [17].

Anticoagulation, as with thromboprophylaxis, is included in the first-line treatment of DVT that involves the use of LMWH rather than intravenous unfractionated heparin. Warfarin, a vitamin K antagonist, is introduced simultaneously, as it is not effective for the first 48 hours of treatment since prothrombin has a half-life of 36 hours. LMWH is continued until the international normalized ratio, achieved by treatment with warfarin, remains in the target range for 2 days. Anticoagulation is continued for at least 3 months depending on the site and extent of the DVT. The treatment may be prolonged to 6-12 months after discussion with the patient. Patients with an underlying familial thrombophilia often require prolonged treatment and may remain on warfarin for life [17].

Thrombolysis tends to be reserved for extensive ilio-femoral DVT or PE with cardio-respiratory compromise. The former requires local catheter-directed delivery of thrombolytic agent, most commonly a tissue plasminogen activator. It is most effective in acute thrombosis (up to 14 days) and complete or partial resolution may be achieved in around 80%. Thombolysis may carry a risk of PE without use of a vena caval filter and is associated with bleeding complications in approximately 10% of patients [17].

Thrombectomy, including surgical thrombectomy and percutaneous mechanical thrombectomy, which has been more popular than catheter-directed thrombolysis recently [12, 23-25], has limited roles and are less commonly used owing to high morbidity and significant re-thrombosis rates [17].

IVC filters may be temporary or permanent. Absolute indications are patients with a contraindication or significant complication related to anticoagulation, recurrent thromboembolic disease on anticoagulation, or an inability to achieve adequate anticoagulation despite patient compliance. Contraindications include complete IVC thrombosis or lack of access to the IVC [17].

The recent American College of Chest Physicians (ACCP) consensus conference on antithrombotic therapy for venous thromboembolic disease has reviewed the existing evidence for the management of patients with ilio-femoral DVT and incorporated recommendations considering treatment algorithm for patients with ilio-femoral DVT including classical anticoagulant therapy for care [26, 27].

Ambulatory Treatment of Ilio-femoral DVT

Ambulatory treatment includes the combination of medical treatment, use of elastic stockings and encouragement of ambulation.

A. Medical Treatment

Medical treatment is composed of use of LMWH (150-175 U, once a day) plus an oral anticoagulant drug (warfarin, coumarin) until international normalized ratio (INR) levels of 2-3 and use of oral anticoagulant drug per se after INR levels of >2. [17].

Administration of LMWHs for 5-10 days as a bridge to oral anticoagulant therapy with vitamin K antagonists for at least 3 months in the treatment of DVT has been confirmed to be as safe and efficient as the conventional anticoagulation by numerous studies and meta-analyses in the literature [3, 28-30].

Enoxaparin, a LMWH, having antithrombotic activity comparable with and theoretically more predictable than unfractionated heparin (UFH) [31, 32] offers an alternative to in-hospital treatment that can be carried out at home, due to its easy administration via subcutaneous (s.c.) route once or twice a day without routine monitoring [3]. Such an option allowing treatment of patients with DVT in an ambulatory setting [33], is considered to be cost-effective, reducing both healthcare costs and hospital length of stay [34, 35] as well as more comfortable for the patients by alleviating pain, improving the quality of life, and lowering the rate of PTS [36, 37].

ACCP Evidence-Based Clinical Practice Guidelines on Antithrombotic and Thrombolytic Therapy; in patients with acute DVT, initial treatment with LMWH (s.c., once or twice daily) for at least 5 days until the INR is >2.0 for 24 h (Grade 1C) has been recommended as an outpatient therapy (Grade 1C) as well as early ambulation in preference to initial bed rest (Grade 1A) [38].

Traditionally, systemic intravenous UFH has been undertaken for 5 days, during which time oral anticoagulation with vitamin K antagonists (usually warfarin) is instituted. INRs therapeutic for 2 consecutive days are usually recommended before stopping heparin [39]. However, due to the need for intravenous administration, the need for frequent partial thromboplastin time monitoring, as well as the bleeding risks of UFH, LMWH has been advanced as the primary therapy for VTE [12].

B. Below-Knee Elastic Stockings (40 mmHg) Starting from the First Day

Graduated compression stockings (GCSs) exert graded pressure from distal to proximal regions of the leg, increasing blood velocity and promoting venous return.

While being suggested in several studies that have challenged the evidence on preferential use of thigh-length stockings, below-knee stockings were shown to be effective in significantly reducing the rate of proximal and calf DVT [40] by relieving venous pump via muscular contraction [41] and reducing the cross-sectional area of the veins and, as a result, increasing the velocity of blood flow in the limb [12] and being helpful in the prevention of edema [41]. Accordingly, any compression above the tibial plateau was shown to have no added benefit over below-knee compression, in relation to preventing venous stasis and increasing the compression at the thigh was reported to be likely to compromise performance further down the leg thus making a case for the preferential choice of below-knee stockings in non-bedridden patients [40].

In accordance with suggestions concerning the use of compression stockings for at least one year and better results indicated for 2-year long treatment [41, 42], compression therapy has become routine for many patients, . This may partly be due to pain or at least swelling tendency, if compression therapy was stopped. Even if follow-up patients who did not wear compression stockings at all and patients with irregular compression therapy did not develop more severe sequela than patients with regular compression therapy, patients who were wearing compression stockings on a regular basis were absent from clinical relevant PTS more often than patients without regular compression therapy [18].

Since compression therapy was shown to be useful also in primary thromboprophylaxis, compression therapy will remain the basic management for patients with chronic venous disorders of the legs [18, 42, 43].

C. Ambulatory Activity (Walking)

There is clear evidence that regular physical activity contributes to the primary and secondary prevention of several chronic diseases such as cardiovascular disease, diabetes and osteoporosis, and is associated with a reduced risk of premature death and improves quality of life [44]. In addition, many patients with DVT and PTS are eager to resume physical activity and seek information about when an exercise program can be restarted and at what intensity [45].

Based on the results of four randomized controlled trials [46-49], there is strong prospective evidence that early walking does not increase the risk of PE in the days after diagnosis and initiation of anticoagulant therapy for DVT [45]. A previous systematic review that included three of the four trials found similar results [50].

Also, high quality evidence from randomized trials showing that home treatment of DVT with anticoagulants is effective and no more liable to complications than hospital treatment [51, 52] and further supports the safety of resuming walking activity early after diagnosis and initiation of treatment for DVT [45].

A tendency for higher levels of physical activity one month after DVT to be associated with less severe post-thrombotic symptoms three months later suggests that increasing physical activity may reduce symptoms of the PTS [53]. As regular exercise has been shown to be beneficial in patients with arterial insufficiency [54, 55], and as there may be an overlap in the mechanisms of leg discomfort that occur in patients with chronic venous and chronic arterial insufficiency, including hypoxic damage to the calf muscle with resultant muscle fiber necrosis, there is the potential for exercise training to help prevent, or treat, the PTS [45].

Current evidence indicates that early walking may be encouraged in patients with acute DVT and that a previous DVT is not a contraindication to regular exercise [45]. Walking additional to good compression does not increase the risk of PE, while significantly decreasing the incidence and severity of pain and swelling after DVT [46, 56].

It is recommended that once patients are therapeutic on anticoagulants they ambulate while wearing compression stockings. The use of strong compression and early ambulation after DVT treatment is initiated can significantly reduce the long-term morbidity of pain and swelling resulting from the DVT and carries a 1A level of evidence [46, 57].

D. Duration of the Treatment

In fact, while the basic treatment of 3 months is acceptable, 5% risk of recurrence even in the most benign cases indicates that the treatment must be continued for 6 months to 1 year in patients with lack of risk factors [58].

The risk of recurrence after discontinuation of anticoagulant therapy is low in patients with transient risk factors (recent surgery, major trauma, prolonged immobilization, pregnancy, puerperium, use of oral contraceptives or hormone replacement therapy) [59-61]. In contrast, patients with persistent risk factors such as cancer, history of VTE and thrombophilia, and patients with idiopathic VTE suffer a high risk of recurrent events up to 20–30% within 5 years [59-62]. Cancer and previous VTE as well as the extension of the thrombus have been identified as independent predictors of recurrence [59, 63, 64].

Since the optimum duration of secondary prophylaxis in patients with VTE is still a matter of debate, the clinical relevance might be the chance for individual adaptation of the duration of long-term anticoagulant therapy to withhold recurrence [64].

Therefore, it is reasonable to inform the patient about the duration of the treatment and to have a consensus on prolonged durations.

The lower extremity venous segments show different proportions of occlusion, partial recanalization, and total recanalization. Calf veins show more rapid recanalization than proximal veins regardless of the involvement in proximal veins [17].

Accordingly, the duration of anticoagulation has been suggested to be longer in patients with proximal DVT than in those with distal DVT [65]. Previous studies revealed that oral anticoagulant is indicated for 3 months or more in patients with proximal DVT [66], for 6 months or more in those with proximal DVT in whom reversible cause cannot be identified, and for 3 months weeks in those with symptomatic calf vein DVT [62].

In fact, patients with hypercoagulability syndrome may need life-long treatment depending on the type of genetic mutation. In patients with a double gene or homozygous mutation recurrence, life-long therapy is indicated since recurrence of 50% has been reported otherwise. In patients with a single recessive mutation, the suggested treatment is 3 to 6 months.

For the prevention of PTS, regardless of the duration of anticoagulant therapy, use of elastic stockings is recommended at least for a year, even up to 2 years in recent publications [12, 40].

As a matter of fact, the curing of the disease occurs within a short period of time but the duration of treatment is crucial to prevent the recurrence.

E. Treatment in Special Patient Populations

In patients with malignancies, evidence of DVT and pulmonary emboli is an indicator of poor prognosis. Pulmonary embolus is the leading cause of death in these patients in case of treatment failure. While using LMWH in 150-175 U once a day and 100 U twice a day was shown to have similar efficacy, the first has been preferred in the daily practice and the latter is preferred in pregnancy during which oral anticoagulant are forbidden due to marked teratogenic effects. Coumadin is prescribed during the breast feeding period since it does not pass into the milk [67].

What Recent TROMBOTEK Trial Adds to Relevant Data on DVT Treatment?

American College of Chest Physicians (ACCP) consensus conference section stated that "there is no evidence that supports the use of thrombolytic agents for the initial treatment of DVT." They recommended against the routine use of catheter-directed thrombolysis (Grade 1C) and indicated that thrombolytic therapy be confined to patients requiring limb salvage (Grade 2C) [51].

Although DVT treatment has been practiced in accordance with ACCP and National Institute for Health and Clinical Excellence (NICE) guidelines [68] in general, feasibility of more invasive techniques including mechanic-thrombolytic treatment that aimed at reducing thrombus burden by means of the recent improvements in operative technique as well as catheter based technology [69] has gained increasing interest in the last decade [15] with the help of significant efforts to increase its popularity including declaration of its lower morbidity and mortality [12, 69].

A spectrum of evidence supporting a strategy of thrombus removal in patients with acute DVT has been published in recent years indicating that patients with extensive DVT, especially those with ilio-femoral thrombosis, will have severe post-thrombotic morbidity if treated with anticoagulation alone. Data is available from experimental observations in animal models, long-term follow-up studies in patients with acute DVT treated with anticoagulation alone, clinical reports of large patient series and randomized trials [12].

The aggregate data overwhelmingly demonstrates that patency can be restored, vein wall and valvular function can be maintained, and post-thrombotic morbidity can be reduced if thrombus is successfully eliminated via aggressive methods and long-term therapeutic anticoagulation maintained to avoid re-thrombosis [12].

The result is the consideration of treatment strategies of thrombus removal including systemic thrombolysis, intra-thrombus catheter-directed thrombolysis, contemporary venous thrombectomy and pharmacomechanical thrombolysis [69] as the far most effective option offering patients the best long-term outcome in the treatment of DVT especially for the thrombosis in the major (ilio-femoral) veins [5].

Previous studies have shown that the time to complete recanalization is considered to be important in the determination of the development of venous valvular reflux [22].

Accordingly, while standard treatment of DVTs via anticoagulation with LMWH or UFH, followed by long-term therapy with vitamin K antagonists, such as warfarin has been shown to effectively reduce the risk of thrombus propagation or recurrence, PE and death, some clinicians believe that anticoagulants have little impact on reducing thrombus size in the short-term, being ineffective in the management of phlegmasia caerulea dolens (PCD) [15]. Besides, both systemic and catheter-directed thrombolysis are considered superior to conventional therapy in clinical practice in relation to significance of rapid thrombolysis in preserving valve function [7].

Furthermore, due to their inability to cause thrombus dissolution, failure to prevent the development of post-thrombotic limb syndrome was suspected in the long-term in many patiens under anticoagulant therapy per se [15].

In this regard, achievement of clot removal via much slower re-canalization process during ambulatory treatment has been accused for the increased risk of PTS (>50%), venous ulcer development (15%) and venous hypertension (95%) as well as significantly disturbed quality of life in patients under the ambulatory treatment [70, 71]. However, all of these findings concerning superiority of thrombolytic treatment to conservative treatment [5] rely on reports published 25-30 years ago when patients were usually treated with UFH in the hospital without compression stockings, enough ambulation and optimal INR follow-up [70, 72].

Whereas early studies showed high prevalence of PTS with conventional treatment of DVT, recent studies show that the prevalence of this disease has decreased due to better therapeutic strategies (i.e. faster diagnosis, intermediate onset of acute therapy and improved monitoring of oral anticoagulant therapy and consequent compression therapy) [18]. Besides, despite the removal of obstruction in the veins and the lesser risk of PTS complication having been accounted for the superiority of thrombolytic treatment, PTS sequel related to this so-called "most effective" treatment seems to reach 15-40% [73].

As a matter of fact, venous thrombectomy and systemic thrombolysis was performed experimentally for many years, however, their true value was never convincingly proven [73] and the need for long-term follow-up studies after thrombolysis has been documented to determine whether improved thrombus resolution translates to better functional outcome and reduced post-thrombotic morbidity [15, 73, 74].

Notably, in a recent randomized trial, the operated group (venous thrombectomy) was reported to have better outcome than the group treated with anticoagulation whereas none of the two groups did very well in the long run [75].

Therefore, owing to significant alterations since the 1990s, including the entrance of novel LMWHs into the market, publications considering efficacy of 3-month LMWH even without oral anticoagulant therapy, more effective and careful use of class II stockings and encouragement of ambulation in the clinical practice, it does not seem reasonable to evaluate the efficacy of ambulatory treatment with respect to data obtained as long as 20 years ago.

On the other hand, although ACCP consensus conference section stated that "there is no evidence that supports the use of thrombolytic agents for the initial treatment of DVT''; the use of stockings plus once daily enoxaparin seem to be subject of a limited number of recent studies [51].

Besides, while treatment of DVT at home with one or two daily doses of LMWH
has been shown to be as effective and safe as in-hospital intravenous (i.v.) UFH [30], few studies have examined the long-term outcomes of a once-daily regimen of LMWH given at home [76].

Accordingly, indicating the significant change in the history of ambulatory treatment history in the past 20 years, with an acknowledgment considering quality of life and successfully managed 18-month follow up, the TROMBOTEK trial by Kurtoglu et al [77] provides excellent evidence that the tools are currently available to manage acute DVT patients with excellent early and long-term outcomes [78].

The TROMBOTEK trial is novel and important, not because it confirms that LMWH transitioning to a vitamin K antagonist is safe and effective but rather because it brings to light that a well-applied, comprehensive, multimodality therapy is highly effective for preventing VTE recurrence and preventing major post-thrombotic morbidity. Unlike many trials that evaluate a single variable intervention, this trial evaluated the "whole package" of evidence-based DVT treatment, with excellent patient follow-up [77, 78].

This trial mimics, in part, several studies showing efficacy of multimodality intensive diabetes therapy, although there was no separate control group in the current study. The primary outcomes were excellent, with a 3.3% VTE recurrence rate, 0.4% PE rate, and 0.7% venous ulceration at 18 months. Safety was also excellent, with a major bleeding rate of 1.6% and an adverse event rate of about 10%. Both of these measures rival prior larger trial end point efficacy [77, 78].

A primary risk for PTS is recurrent DVT and a greater extent of DVT. Although the incidence of CEAP (clinical, etiologic, anatomic and pathophysiologic) C4 through C6 disease (more severe PTS) was low in this study, it should be known that the best measure for PTS is the Villalta score, and thus this study may underestimate some of the disability related to the patient's DVT [78, 79]. Nevertheless, while a lack of Villalta, which is one of the most important scoring systems used for PTS, is a significant limitation of the study, compensating for this limitation, CEAP findings seem to enable symptomatic analysis amongst patients during the course of the study.

Regardless, the low rate of PTS may be because therapeutic anticoagulation compliance rates were high (80%) and those patients with an unprovoked DVT were very low; both of these factors are associated with an increased risk of PTS [80]. Nonetheless, the large number of patients in this study with an ilio-femoral DVT, a significant risk factor for PTS, underscores the effectiveness of this multimodality therapy; that is, most of these ilio-femoral segments recanalized over time [78].

Notably, our findings in the TROMBOTEK trial seem to challenge the wide application of expensive and invasive pharmaco-mechanical therapy for all DVT patients. Similarly, in a recent trial, prolonged LMWH therapy was reported to be associated with a significant reduction in PTS compared with standard anticoagulation [58].

Therefore, when compared to the old literature [70, 72] on conservative approach in DVT treatment, the main differences in the THROMBOTEK trial were the administration of once-a-day LMWH (enoxaparin) therapy, class II compression stockings for at least one year, intense ambulation at home and the sufficient evidence against inclusion of all patients under a single model, while most of the study population was composed of post-operative DVT patients.

LMWHs administered subcutaneously once or twice daily have been reported to be as safe and effective as intravenous UFH in the treatment of VTE in large, well-established, prospective, multicenter trials [3, 28-30, 81, 82]. VTE treatment was associated in the TROMBOTEK trial with a significant reduction in the incidence of symptoms, circumference of the thrombotic leg, D-dimer scores and marked improvement of recanalization ratios for occluded veins [77].

Conservative treatment has been accused for the slower process of recanalization especially in ilio-femoral veins resulting in 30% of obstructions to be permanent even after recanalization. In this regard, thrombolytic treatment has been preferred in most instances due to rapid removel of clot. However, TROMBOTEK data has shown complete recanalization in more than 80% of iliac veins in ultrasonographic evaluations during follow up for 18 months under ambulatory treatment. Moreover, indicating similar lack of efficacy in distal veins, lesser recanalization in distal (infrainguinal) veins was reported in the TROMBOTEK trial, alike to studies concerning thrombolytic treatment.

Hence, in contrast to statements indicating that classical anticoagulant therapy has low efficacy in recanalization of the ilio-femoral vein and more common observation of post-thrombotic chronic venous insufficiency, leg ulceration and venous claudication as well as a 2.6-fold higher risk of recurrence [69] in patients with ilio-femoral DVT treated with anticoagulation alone; our results concerning early obtainment and following maintenance of complete recanalization ratio in the ilio-femoral vein by means of enoxparine plus warfarin therapy accompanied with graduated compression stockings seems promising [15, 83]. However, the possible role of high prevalence of provoked DVT among our patients in this success needs further clarification.

Notably, venous ulcer incidence of %0.07 given in the TROMBOTEK population under the ambulatory treatment seems to be the most significant proof against the considerations indicating inefficacy of ambulatory treatment based on high risk of venous risk reaching 15% by ambulatory treatment based on old-literature.

For these reasons, we declare conventional conservative treatment to be the most ideal alternative carrying a 1A level of evidence comparable to thrombolytic treatment.

In fact, not examined by the TROMBOTEK trial is likely cost-saving by ambulatory treatment resulting from outpatient treatment as the primary mode, thus eliminating the need for laboratory draws (activated partial thromboplastin time) and an inpatient stay as well as significant reduction in the work force loss.

Conclusion

As with so many other diseases, systems to ensure comprehensive treatment for a disease from start to finish are critical and should be an area of national healthcare priority. The gap in so many of these diseases is not the tools, but the consistent application of these tools in a timely and appropriate manner [82].

Based on results of TROMBOTEK trial, ambulatory treatment with enoxaparin plus warfarin accompanied with graduated compression stockings seem to be effective in symptomatic healing as well as clinical improvement by reducing thrombus formation/organization at all levels of lower limb venous system in DVT without a significant major bleeding risk. A conventional conservative treatment having a level of evidence 1A may seem to have comparable and even preferable results in terms of better cost-effectiveness to thrombolytic treatment recommended in recent studies especially for ilio-femoral DVT. Further randomized controlled trials are needed to confirm these conclusions.

Recent improvements in the anticoagulant drug industry and a market-enabled shift from the use of classical heparin to LMWH/ultra-low-molecular weight heparin (ULMWH) as well as a shift from oral anticoagulant warfarin to novel molecules in the clinical practice. In fact, a conduction of investigations considering these so far novel agents in comparison to more recently developed ones in the future seems critical to prevent similar inter-therapeutic conflicts.

References

[1]   Deitcher, S.R., Carman, T.L. Deep venous thrombosis and pulmonary embolism. *Curr. Treat. Options. Cardiovasc. Med.* 2002; 4: 223-38.

[2]   Vieira, L.M., Dusse, L.M., Fernandes, A.P., Martins-Filho, O.A., de Bastos, M., Ferreira, M.F., et al. Monocytes and plasma tissue factor levels in normal individuals and patients with deep venous thrombosis of the lower limbs: potential diagnostic tools? *Thromb. Res.* 2007; 119(2): 157-65.

[3]   Shapiro, N.I., Spear, J., Sheehy, S., Brown, J., Edlow, J.A. Barriers to the use of outpatient enoxaparin therapy in patients with deep venous thrombosis. *Am. J. Emerg. Med.* 2005; 23(1): 30-4.

[4]   Kurtoglu, M. Deep Vein Thrombosis. In: Ertekin, C., Taviloglu, K., Guloglu, R., Kurtoğlu, M., editors. Trauma. 1st ed.İstanbul Medikal Yayıncılık p. 1343-57, 2005.

[5]   Comerota, A.J., Paolini, D. Treatment of acute ilio-femoral deep venous thrombosis: a strategy of thrombus removal. *Eur. J. Vasc. Endovasc. Surg.* 2007; 33(3): 351-60.

[6]   Agnelli, G., Verso, M., Ageno, W., Imberti, D., Moia, M., Palareti, G., Rossi, R., Pistelli, R; MASTER investigators. The MASTER registry on venous thromboembolism: description of the study cohort. *Thromb. Res.* 2008; 121(5): 605-10.

[7]   Laiho, M.K., Oinonen, A., Sugano, N., Harjola, V.P., Lehtola, A.L., Roth, W.D., Keto, P.E., Lepäntalo, M. Preservation of venous valve function after catheter-directed and systemic thrombolysis for deep venous thrombosis. *Eur. J. Vasc. Endovasc. Surg.* 2004; 28(4): 391-6.

[8]   Ginsberg, J.S. Management of venous thromboembolism. *N. Engl. J. Med.* 1996; 335: 1816-1828.

[9]   Hyers, T.M., Hull, R.D., Weg, G.J. Antithrombotic therapy for venous thromboembolic disease. *Chest.*1998; 114: 561S-578S.

[10] Hirsh, J., Hoak, J. Management of deep vein thrombosis and pulmonary embolism. A statement for healthcare professionals. *Circulation.* 1996; 93: 2212-2245.

[11] Pinede, L., Ninet, J., Duhaut, P., Chabaud, S., Demolombe-Rague, S., Durieu, I., Nony, P., Sanson, C., Boissel, J.P. Investigators of the "Durée Optimale du Traitement AntiVitamines K" (DOTAVK) Study. Comparison of 3 and 6 months of oral anticoagulant therapy after a first episode of proximal deep vein thrombosis or pulmonary embolism and comparison of 6 and 12 weeks of therapy after isolated calf deep vein thrombosis. *Circulation.* 2001; 103(20): 2453-60.

[12] Wakefield, T.W., Caprini, J., Comerota, A.J. Thromboembolic diseases. *Curr. Probl. Surg.* 2008; 45(12): 844-99.

[13] Meissner, M.H., Wakefield, T.W., Ascher, E., Caprini, J.A., Comerota, A.J., Eklof, B., et al. Acute venous disease: venous thrombosis and venous trauma. *J. Vasc. Surg.* 2007; 46(Suppl. S): 25-53.

[14] Menon, J., Hamilton, G. Deep venous thrombosis. *Surgery.* 2007; 25: 323-6.

[15] Gogalniceanu, P., Johnston, C.J., Khalid, U., Holt, P.J., Hincliffe, R., Loftus, I.M., Thompson, M.M. Indications for thrombolysis in deep venous thrombosis. *Eur. J. Vasc. Endovasc. Surg.* 2009; 38(2): 192-8.

[16] Fowkes, F.J., Price, J.F., Fowkes, F.G. Incidence of diagnosed deep vein thrombosis in the general population. *Eur. J. Vasc. Endovasc. Surg.* 2003; 25: 1-5.

[17] Winterborn, R., Smith, F. Deep venous thrombosis. *Surgery.* 2009; 27(8): 326-330.

[18] Ziegler, S., Schillinger, M., Maca, T.H., Minar, E. Post-thrombotic syndrome after primary event of deep venous thrombosis 10 to 20 years ago. *Thromb. Res.* 2001; 101(2): 23-33.

[19] Epstein, N.E. A review of the risks and benefits of differing prophylaxis regimens for the treatment of deep venous thrombosis and pulmonary embolism in neurosurgery. *Surg. Neurol.* 2005; 64(4): 295-301.

[20] Geerts, W.H., Pineo, G.F., Heit, J.A., Bergqvist, D., Lassen, M.R., Colwell, C.W., et al. Prevention of Venous Thromboembolism: the Seventh ACCP Conference on Antithrombotic and Thrombolytic Therapy. *Chest.* 2004; 126 (3 suppl): 338S-400S.

[21] Prandoni, P., Lensing, A.W., Prins, M.R. Long-term outcomes after deep venous thrombosis of the lower extremities. *Vasc. Med.* 1998; 3: 57-60.

[22] Yamaki, T., Nozaki, M. Patterns of venous insufficiency after an acute deep vein thrombosis. *J. Am. Coll. Surg.* 2005; 201(2): 231-8.

[23] Lee, K-H., Han, H., Lee, K.J., Yoon, C-S., Kim, S.H., Won, J.Y., et al. Mechanical thrombectomy of acute ilio-femoral deep vein thrombosis with use of an Arrow-Trerotola percutaneous thrombectomy device. *J. Vasc. Interv. Radiol.* 2006; 17: 487-95.

[24] Cynamon, J., Stein, E.G., Dym, R.J., Jagust, M.B., Binkert, C.A., Baum, R.A. A new method of aggressive management of deep vein thrombosis: retrospective study of the power pulse technique. *J. Vasc. Interv. Radiol.* 2006; 17: 1043-9.

[25] Vedantham, S., Vesely, T.M., Sicard, G.A., Brown, D., Rubin, B., Sanchez, L.A., et al. Pharmacomechanical thrombolysis and early stent placement for ilio-femoral deep vein thrombosis. *J. Vasc. Interv. Radiol.* 2004; 15: 565-74.

[26] Guyatt, G.H., Cook, D.J., Jaeschke, R., Pauker, S.G., Schünemann, H.J. Grades of recommendation for anti-thrombotic agents: American College of Chest Physicians Evidence-Based Clinical Practice Guidelines (8th Edition). *Chest.* 2008; 133:123S-31S.

[27] Kearon, C., Kahn, S.R., Agnelli, G., Goldhaber, S.Z., Raskob, G., Comerota, A.J. Antithrombotic Therapy for Venous Thromboembolic Disease: ACCP Evidence- Based Clinical Practice Guidelines (8th Edition). *Chest.* 2008; 133(6 Suppl): 454S-545S.

[28] Bratt, G., Aberg, W., Johansson, M., Törnebohm, E., Granqvist, S., Lockner, D. Two daily subcutaneous injections of fragmin as compared with intravenous standard heparin in the treatment of deep venous thrombosis (DVT). *Thromb. Haemost.* 1990; 64: 506-10.

[29] Simonneau, G., Charbonnier, B., Decousus, H., Planchon, B., Ninet, J., Sie, P., et al. Subcutaneous low molecular-weight heparin compared with continuous intravenous unfractionated heparin in the treatment of proximal deep vein thrombosis. *Arch. Intern. Med.* 1993; 153: 1541-6.

[30] Levine, M., Gent, M., Hirsh, J., Leclerc, J., Anderson, D., Weitz, J., et al. A comparison of low-molecular weight heparin administered primarily at home with unfractionated heparin administered in the hospital for proximal deep-vein thrombosis. *N. Engl. J. Med.*1996; 334: 677-81.

[31] Dawes, J., Bara, L., Billaud, E., Samama, M. Relationship between biological activity and concentration of a low-molecular weight heparin (PK- 10169) and unfractionated heparin after intravenous and subcutaneous administration. *Haemostasis.* 1986; 16(2): 116-22.

[32] Shaieb, M.D., Watson, B.N., Atkinson, R.E. Bleeding complications with enoxaparin for deep venous thrombosis prophylaxis. *J. Arthroplasty.* 1999; 14(4): 432-8.

[33] Wells, P.S. Outpatient treatment of patients with deep vein thrombosis or pulmonary embolism. *Curr. Opin. Pulm. Med.* 2001; 7: 360-4.

[34] Trujillo-Santos, J., Perea-Milla, E., Jiménez-Puente, A., Sánchez-Cantalejo, E., del Toro, J., Grau, E., et al. RIETE Investigators. Bed rest or ambulation in the initial treatment of patients with acute deep vein thrombosis or pulmonary embolism: findings from the RIETE registry. *Chest.* 2005; 127: 1631-41.

[35] Partsch, H., Kechavarz, B., Köhn, H., Mostbeck, A. The effect of mobilization of patients during treatment of thromboembolic disorders with LMWH. *Int. Angiol.* 1997; 16:189-92.

[36] Partsch, H., Kaulich, M., Mayer, W. Immediate mobilization in acute vein thrombosis reduces post-thrombotic syndrome. *Int. Angiol.* 2004; 23: 206-12.

[37] Partsch, H. Bed rest versus ambulation in the initial treatment of patients with proximal deep vein thrombosis. *Curr. Opin. Pulm. Med.* 2002; 8: 389-93.

[38] Hirsh, J., Guyatt, G., Albers, G.W., Harrington, R., Schunemann, H.J. American College of Chest Physicians Evidence-Based Clinical Practice

Guidelines (8th Edition). Antithrombotic and Thrombolytic Therapy 8th Ed: ACCP Guidelines. *Chest.* 2008; 133: 71-105.

[39] Bates, S.M., Ginsberg, J.S. Clinical practice. Treatment of deep vein thrombosis. *N. Engl. J. Med.* 2004; 351: 268-77.

[40] Autar, R. A review of the evidence for the efficacy of Anti-Embolism Stockings (AES) in Venous Thromboembolism (VTE) prevention. *J. Orth. Nurs.* 2009; 13: 41-49.

[41] Partsch, H. Use of Compression Therapy. In Sclerotherapy, 5th ed.- Treatment of Varicose and Telangiectatic Leg Veins. Goldman MP, Guex JJ, Weiss RA, et al. (eds.) 2011, pp123-155.

[42] Partsch, H., Kechavarz, B., Mostbeck, A., Kohn, A. Therapy of deep vein thrombosis with low molecular weight heparin, compression bandage and walking exercise. *Med. Welt.* 1997; 48(2): 84-90.

[43] Brandjes, D.P.M., Buller, H.R., Heijboer, H., Huisman, M.V., de Rijk, M., Jagt, H., Ten Cate, J.W. Randomized trial of effects of compression stockings in patients with symptomatic proximal-vein thrombosis. *Lancet.* 1997; 349: 759-62.

[44] Warburton, D.E.R., Nicol, C.W., Bredin, S.S.D. Health benefits of physical activity: the evidence. *Can. Med. Assoc. J.* 2006; 174: 801-9.

[45] Kahn, S.R., Shrier, I., Kearon, C. Physical activity in patients with deep venous thrombosis: a systematic review. *Thromb. Res.* 2008; 122(6): 763-73.

[46] Aschwanden, M., Labs, K.H., Engel, H., Schwob, A., Jeanneret, C., Mueller-Brand, J., et al. Acute deep vein thrombosis: early mobilization does not increase the frequency of pulmonary embolism. *Thromb. Haemost.* 2001; 85: 42-6.

[47] Schellong, S.M., Schwarz, T., Kropp, J., Prescher, Y., Beuthien-Baumann, B., Daniel, W.G. Bed rest in deep vein thrombosis and the incidence of scintigraphic pulmonary embolism. *Thromb. Haemost.* 1999; 82 (Suppl 1): 127-9.

[48] Blattler, W., Partsch, H. Leg compression and ambulation is better than bed rest for the treatment of acute deep venous thrombosis. *Int. Angiol.* 2003; 22: 393-400.

[49] Junger, M., Diehm, C., Storiko, H., Hach-Wunderle, V., Heidrich, H., Karasch, T., et al. Mobilization versus immobilization in the treatment of acute proximal deep venous thrombosis: a prospective, randomized, open, multicenter trial. *Curr. Med. Res. Opin.* 2006; 22: 593-602.

[50] Trujillo-Santos, A.J., Martos-Perez, F., Perea-Milla, E. Bed rest or early mobilization as treatment of deep vein thrombosis: a systematic review and meta-analysis. *Med. Clin. (Barc).* 2004; 122: 641-7.

[51] Buller, H.R., Agnelli, G., Hull, R.D., Hyers, T.M., Prins, M.H., Raskob, G.E. Antithrombotic therapy for venous thromboembolic disease: the Seventh ACCP Conference on Antithrombotic and Thrombolytic Therapy. *Chest.* 2004; 126: 401S-28S.

[52] Schraibman, I.G., Milne, A.A., Royle, E.M. Home versus in-patient treatment for deep vein thrombosis. *Cochrane. Database. Syst. Rev.* 2001: CD003076.

[53] Shrier, I., Kahn, S.R. Effect of physical activity after recent deep venous thrombosis: a cohort study. *Med. Sci. Sports. Exerc.* 2005; 37: 630-4.

[54] Gardner, A.W., Poehlman, E.T. Exercise rehabilitation programs for the treatment of claudication pain. A meta-analysis. *JAMA.* 1995; 274: 975-80.

[55] Leng, G.C., Fowler, B., Ernst, E. Exercise for intermittent claudication. *Cochrane. Database. Syst. Rev.* 2000: CD000990.

[56] Partsch, H. Ambulation and compression after deep vein thrombosis: dispelling myths. *Semin. Vasc. Surg.* 2005; 18: 148-52.

[57] Prandoni, P., Lensing, A.W., Prins, M.H., Frulla, M., Marchiori, A., Bernardi, E., et al. Below-knee elastic compression stockings to prevent the post-thrombotic syndrome: a randomized, controlled trial. *Ann. Intern. Med.* 2004; 141: 249-56.

[58] Hull, R.D., Pineo, G.F., Brant, R.F., Mah, A.F., Burke, N., Dear, R., et al. Long-term low-molecular-weight heparin versus usual care in proximalvein thrombosis patients with cancer. *Am. J. Med.* 2006; 119: 1062-72.

[59] Hansson, P.O., Sorbo, J., Eriksson, H. Recurrent venous thromboembolism after deep vein thrombosis: incidence and risk factors. *Arch. Intern. Med.*2000; 160(6): 769-74.

[60] Prandoni, P., et al. The long-term clinical course of acute deep venous thrombosis. *Ann Intern Med* 1996; 125(1): 1 -7.

[61] Sudlow, M.F., Campbell, I.A., Angel, J.H., Bentley, P., Fennerty, A.G., Prescott, R.J., Routledge, P.A. Optimum duration of anticoagulation for deep vein thrombosis and pulmonary embolism. Research committee of the British Thoracic Society. *Lancet.* 1992; 340 (8824): 873-6.

[62] Schulman, S., et al. A comparison of six weeks with six months of oral anticoagulant therapy after a first episode of venous thromboembolism. Duration of Anticoagulation Trial Study Group. *N. Engl. J. Med.* 1995; 332(25): 1661- 5.

[63] Ouriel, K., et al. The anatomy of deep venous thrombosis of the lower extremity. *J. Vasc. Surg.* 2000;31(5):895– 900.

[64] Alt, E., Banyai, S., Banyai, M., Koppensteiner, R. Blood rheology in deep venous thrombosis--relation to persistent and transient risk factors. *Thromb. Res.* 2002; 15; 107 (3-4): 101-7.

[65] Hirsh, J., Fuster, V., Ansell, J., Halperin, J.L. American Heart Association/American College of Cardiology Foundation guide to warfarin therapy. *Circulation.* 2003; 107:1692-1711.

[66] Hull, R., Delmore, T., Carter, C., et al. Adjusted subcutaneous heparin versus warfarin sodium in the long-term treatment of venous thrombosis. *N. Engl. J. Med.* 1982; 306: 189-194.

[67] Ulander, V.M., Stenqvist, P., Kaaja, R. Treatment of deep venous thrombosis with low-molecular-weight heparin during pregnancy. *Thromb. Res.* 2002; 106 (1): 13-7.

[68] NICE National Collaborating Centre for Acute Care. Venous thromboembolism: reducing the risk of venous thromboembolism (deep vein thrombosis and pulmonary embolism) in inpatients undergoing surgery. National Institute of Clinical Excellence (NICE) Guidelines. London: NICE. Also available at: http://www.nice.org.uk/ nicemedia/ pdf/VTEFullGuide.pdf; 2007 (accessed).

[69] Comerota, A.J., Gravett, M.H. Ilio-femoral venous thrombosis. *J. Vasc. Surg.* 2007; 46 (5): 1065-76. Review.

[70] Akesson, H., Brudin, L., Dahlstrom, J.A., Eklof, B., Ohlin, P., Plate, G. Venous function assessed during a 5 year period after acute ilio-femoral venous thrombosis treated with anticoagulation. *Eur. J. Vasc. Surg.* 1990; 4 (1): 43-48.

[71] Comerota, A.J. Catheter-directed thrombolysis is the appropriate treatment for ilio-femoral deep venous thrombosis. *Dis. Mon.* 2010; 56 (11): 637-41.

[72] O'Donnell, T.F., Browse, N.L., Burnand, K.G., Thomas, M.L. The socioeconomic effects of an ilio-femoral venous thrombosis. *J. Surg. Res.* 1977; 22(5): 483-488.

[73] Sillesen, H., Just, S., Jørgensen, M., Baekgaard, N. Catheter-directed thrombolysis for treatment of ilio-femoral deep venous thrombosis is durable, preserves venous valve function and may prevent chronic venous insufficiency. *Eur. J. Vasc. Endovasc. Surg.* 2005; 30(5): 556-62.

[74] Motaganahalli, R., Dalsing, M.C. Deep venous interventions. In: Fast Facts: Vascular and Endovascular Surgery Highlights 2009-10. By Alun H. Davies (editor), Health Press, UK, pp11-15.

[75] Plate, G., Akesson, H., Einarsson, E., Ohlin, P., Eklof, B. Long-term results of venous throm-bectomy combined with temporary arteriovenous fistula. *Eur. J. Vasc. Surg.* 1990; 4: 483-489.

[76] Ramacciotti, E., Araújo, G.R., Lastoria, S., Maffei, F.H., Karaoglan de Moura, L., Michaelis, Wet., al. CLETRAT Investigators. An open-label, comparative study of the efficacy and safety of once-daily dose of enoxaparin versus unfractionated heparin in the treatment of proximal lower limb deep-vein thrombosis. *Thromb. Res.* 2004; 114(3): 149-53.

[77] Kurtoglu, M., Koksoy, C., Hasan, E., Akcalı, Y., Karabay, O., Filizcan, U.; TROMBOTEK Study Group. Long-term efficacy and safety of once-daily enoxaparin plus warfarin for the outpatient ambulatory treatment of lower-limb deep vein thrombosis in the TROMBOTEK trial. *J. Vasc. Surg.* 2010; 52(5): 1262-70.

[78] Henke, PK. Invited commentary on "Long-term efficacy and safety of once-daily enoxaparin plus warfarin for the outpatient ambulatory treatment of lower-limb deep vein thrombosis in the TROMBOTEK trial". *J. Vasc. Surg.* 2010; 52(5): 1270-71.

[79] Kahn, S.R., Partsch, H., Vedantham, S., Prandoni, P., Kearon, C. Definition of post-thrombotic syndrome of the leg for use in clinical investigations: a recommendation for standardization. *J. Thromb. Haemost.* 2009; 7: 879-83.

[80] Kahn, S.R., Shrier, I., Julian, J.A., Ducruet, T., Arsenault, L., Miron, M.J., et al. Determinants and time course of the post-thrombotic syndrome after acute deep venous thrombosis. *Ann. Intern. Med.* 2008; 149: 698-707.

[81] Koopman, M.M., Prandoni, P., Piovella, F., Ockelford, P.A., Brandjes, D..P, van der Meer, J., et al. Treatment of venous thrombosis with intravenous unfractionated heparin administered in the hospital as compared with subcutaneous low-molecular-weight heparin administered at home. The Tasman Study Group. *N. Engl. J. Med.* 1996; 334: 682-7.

[82] Merli, G., Spiro, T.E., Olsson, C.G., Abildgaard, U., Davidson, B.L., Eldor, A., et al. Enoxaparin Clinical Trial Group. Subcutaneous enoxaparin once or twice daily compared with intravenous unfractionated heparin for treatment of venous thromboembolic disease. *Ann. Intern. Med.* 2001; 134(3): 191-202.

[83] Gutt, C.N., Oniu, T., Wolkener, F., Mehrabi, A., Mistry, S., Büchler, M.W. Prophylaxis and treatment of deep vein thrombosis in general surgery. *Am. J. Surg.* 2005; 189(1): 14-22.

In: Deep Vein Thrombosis
Editor: Takashi Yamaki

ISBN: 978-1-62257-519-0
© 2013 Nova Science Publishers, Inc.

Chapter 6

Management of Deep Vein Thrombosis with Oral Vitamin K Antagonist

Pinjala Ramakrishna[*]
Department of Vascular Surgery,
Nizam's Institute of Medical Sciences, India

Abstract

Oral vitamin K antagonist therapy is useful for prevention and treatment of thromboembolic disease. The fear of medication errors and medication related adverse events limit the appropriate use of oral vitamin k antagonist therapy. The beneficial effectiveness of oral vitamin K antagonist therapy depends on the adequate dose and its long term management. Acenocoumarol and warfarin are the commonly used vitamin K antagonists (VKAs) in our practice. Long term management (6 months) of the DVT patients with vitamin K antagonists has increased in recent years with improvement in the diagnostic methods of DVT detection and increasing age of the population. The pharmacokinetic and pharmacodynamic properties of the vitamin K antagonists along with the narrow therapeutic range make the management of oral anticoagulation

[*] Correspondence to: Professor Pinjala Ramakrishna, MS., FRCSEd, FICS. Department of Vascular Surgery, Nizam's Institute of Medical Sciences, Hyderabad, AP, India, Telephone: +91-40-23317115. E-mail:pinjala@hotmail.com.

for thromboembolic complications complex. Patients receiving oral anticoagulants are likely to attend emergency department due to bleeding from the medication errors. So, this is a serious concern in many countries and one would like to avoid the medication errors by maintaining the high quality of anticoagulation in DVT patients. During the initiation of oral anticoagulation therapy injection of heparin and oral anticoagulants are overlapped till the therapeutic INR values are achieved with the vitamin K antagonists. This overlap is maintained till two consecutive INR values are above 2.0. We generally start oral anticoagulation with 5mgs of tablet warfarin or 4mgs of tablet Acitrom as the higher doses are known to precipitate early hemorrhages. In the elderly people, undernourished, heart failure, liver disease and postoperative patients the anticoagulation is initiated with smaller doses (<5 mgs) due to the fear of bleeding. CYP2C9 is the principal enzyme to metabolize the oral anticoagulants and polymorphisms of the gene coding CYP2C9 can result in abnormalities. Recent studies are showing the advantages of pharmacogenetic based dosing to overcome these abnormalities, but it is not yet widely accepted or recommended. The warfarin inhibits the vitamin K oxide reductase complex (VKORC) and mutation of the genes coding this enzyme complex (VKORC1) can increase the sensitivity or resistance to warfarin inhibition. The adequate therapeutic dose to maintain INR shows variability due to these mutations. The therapeutic anticoagulation (INR>2) should be maintained to get maximum benefit. That means the time in therapeutic range (TTR) correlates with the clinical outcomes of hemorrhage and thrombosis. Increased TTR has also been associated with decreased mortality. INR test is performed at regular intervals of 7-14 days depending on the stable dose response in a given patient. Management of non-therapeutic INR is difficult in patients with complex life styles and variable dietary habits. Non-compliance and concomitant medications makes this more difficult to manage and maintain the therapeutic INRs. The target therapeutic INRs can be achieved by adjusting the warfarin doses with up or down increments of 5-20% and frequent monitoring. When the INR is between 4-10 without bleeding it is better to stop the medication and monitor the INR daily and restart with the reduced weekly dose of INR after it has fallen to the therapeutic range. Abnormally elevated INRs with or without bleeding would need attention and careful follow up adjustment of doses. We are cautious in correcting the abnormally high INRs associated with bleeding with Vitamin K injections which can increase the vitamin K resistance to warfarin later. Correction dose requirements are dependent on age, race, BMI, concomitant medications, co-morbidities and gene mutations. Systematic reviews of the patients on warfarin have shown bleeding rates of 8.9% per patient year in first 3 months, only 2.5% after 3 months of initiation of anticoagulation therapy. When patients are actively bleeding while they are on oral vitamin K antagonists one would target rapid lowering of the INRs with infusion of fresh frozen plasma (FFP), Prothrombin concentrates or recombinant factor VIIa along with injection vitamin K to facilitate the endogenous coagulation factor production. Quality patient education is necessary to achieve the safe and effective oral anticoagulation with Vitamin K antagonists under the supervision of the treating teams. It is indeed a challenge for the teams providing the oral anticoagulation therapies to prevent the recurrent thrombosis and thromboembolism in deep vein thrombosis in patients in many countries through quality education of patients to achieve the maximum time in therapeutic range.

Introduction

Venous thrombosis is a common disease with a yearly incidence of around one case per 1000 person-years [1] and it is often missed in the early stages. Venous thrombosis is known to recur frequently. Recurrence can be prevented or reduced by appropriate use of anticoagulants but this is associated with risk of bleeding. Assessment of the risk of recurrence is important to balance the risks and benefits of anticoagulation treatment. The risk of major bleeding in patients who are receiving anticoagulation treatment is around 3% per year in clinical trials and is higher in routine practice [2]. The case-fatality rate of fatal bleeding in patients who were given anticoagulant treatment was reported to be as high as 11·3%.

Anticoagulants continue to remain as the mainstay of treatment of venous thromboembolism (VTE). The study by Barritt and Jordan [3] established the role of anticoagulants in venous thromboembolism. In this study they randomized 35 patients with clinically diagnosed with pulmonary embolism (PE) to treatment with heparin or to no treatment. There were no fatalities in the heparin-treated group. In contrast, 25% of those untreated died of autopsy-proven PE. This study suggested that rapid anticoagulation is necessary to minimize the risk of thrombus extension and PE in patients with venous thromboembolism. This concept was also supported by the placebo-controlled study of Brandjes et al [4] which randomized 120 patients with proximal DVT to treatment with heparin plus a vitamin K antagonist or to a vitamin K antagonist alone. The study was stopped prematurely because the rate of symptomatic recurrent VTE was lower in those given heparin plus a vitamin K antagonist than in those treated only with a vitamin K antagonist. After initial treatment with heparin or LMWH, ongoing anticoagulant therapy is needed to prevent recurrent VTE. [5] Extended therapy usually involves administration of a vitamin K antagonist and the newer studies show that LMWH may be a better choice in cancer patients with venous thromboembolism.

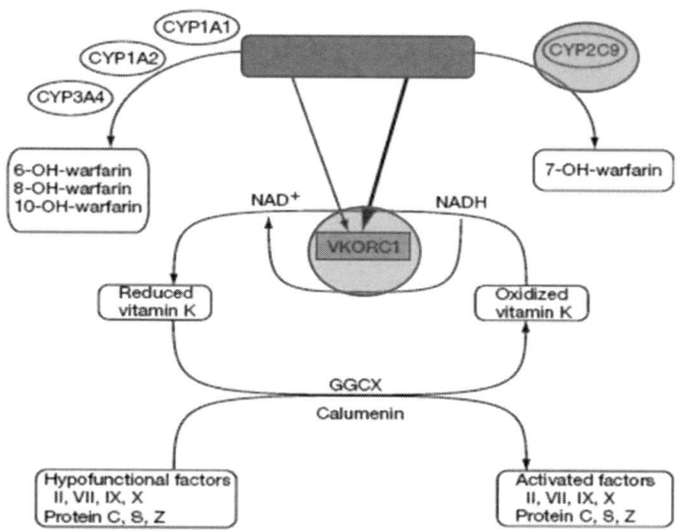

Figure 1. Pharmcogenomics and Vitamin K antagonits.

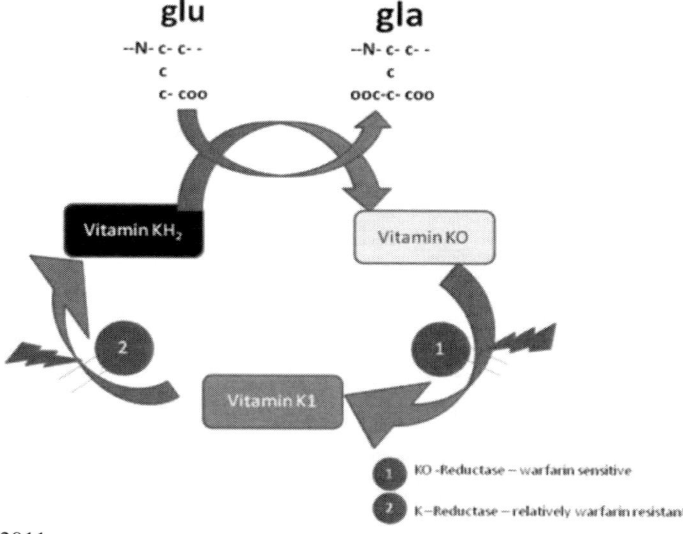

Pinjala `2011.

Figure 2. Mechanism of action of Vitamin K antagonist.

Usually a 3-month course of anticoagulant treatment is adequate for patients with VTE precipitated by a transient risk factor, such as surgery. More extended therapy is needed in patients with unprovoked VTE. Long-term anticoagulation therapy is problematic because vitamin K antagonists require regular monitoring. Routine coagulation monitoring is essential to ensure that a good therapeutic response is obtained. The vitamin K antagonists have a narrow therapeutic window. The sub-therapeutic dose responses do not reduce the risk of thrombosis and excessive anticoagulation increases the risk of bleeding.

Interactions with a range of drugs can reduce or enhance the anticoagulant effects of vitamin K antagonists. Similarly variable intake of foods containing vitamin K can alter the effects. Genetically determined polymorphisms in the cytochrome P4502C9 (CYP2C9) enzyme can alter the metabolism of vitamin K antagonists (see Figure 1). In spite of regular monitoring of anticoagulation, patients who are taking vitamin K antagonists have a therapeutic anticoagulant response less than half the time that increases the risk for complications.

Approximately 15 to 20 per 1000 subjects in the western world use vitamin K antagonists. [6]. It was also estimated that more than 1 million residents in United Kingdom take warfarin. The search for better drugs which are safer and simpler for the patients to accept and prevent the recurrent venous thromboembolic complications is unending.

The cost of preventing death from pulmonary embolism has been derived from several prophylactic measures after general surgery and orthopedic hip surgery. In general surgery, Salzman et al estimated the cost of preventing one fatal pulmonary embolism through the use of low dose heparin has been estimated at US$900. [7] Similarly Paiement GD et al estimated the analogous cost for 3 months warfarin Thromboprophylaxis after hip replacement as US$1000 [8]. These values may vary from country to country depending on the drug cost and care costs. In India, the cost of therapy with oral anticoagulants may be low but the cost of managing bleeding due to lack of regular monitoring of INR will be much higher.

Mechanism of Action of Vitamin K Antagonists – as Anticoagulants

Cyclical inter conversion of the vitamin K and its 2, 3 epoxide (vitamin K epoxide) is essential for the carboxylation of the glutamate residues on

N-terminal regions of the vitamin K dependent proteins. The coagulation factors II, VII, IX and X need carboxylation for their biological activity. Vitamin K antagonists inhibit this cyclical interconversion of the vitamin K and results in hepatic production of partially carboxylated or decarboxylated proteins with reduced procoagulant activity. These vitamin antagonists also inhibit the carboxylation of the Protein C, Protein S and therefore they have the potential to produce procoagulant effect during the initiation phase. The carboxylation which occurs in the presence of calcium ions produces conformational changes in the coagulation proteins and promotes binding to the cofactors. Carboxylation needs reduced form of vitamin K (vitamin KH_2), molecular oxygen and carbon dioxide and is linked to the oxidation of vitamin KH_2 to vitamin K epoxide. Vitamin K is then recycled to vitamin KH_2 through two reductase steps. The first of these reductase steps (vitamin K epoxide to vitamin K1) is sensitive to the vitamin K antagonists and the 2nd is relatively insensitive to the vitamin K antagonists (vitamin K1 to vitamin KH_2). The Vitamin K1 supplementation can counter the effects of the vitamin K antagonists bypassing the 1st reductase step. These vitamin K antagonists can also interfere with the carboxylation of the proteins synthesized during the bone development and that may produce fetal bone abnormalities if the mothers are treated with these drugs during pregnancy.

Pharmacodynamics and Pharmacokinetics of Warfarin (Vitamin K Antagonist)

The drug, Warfarin is a mixture of two forms (R and S forms) which are optically active isomers. It can get easily absorbed from the GI tract and so it has high bioavailability. Maximum blood levels are reached within 90 minutes after ingestion. The racemic warfarin has a half-life of 36 to 42 hours and it is bound to albumin while circulating in the blood and later gets accumulated in the liver. Hereditary resistance to Warfarin occurs in the rats as well as in human beings. Patients with genetic warfarin resistance may require higher doses of warfarin to achieve the therapeutic level of anticoagulation. In such cases the dose requirement many be 5 fold to 20 fold higher than the average doses. Mutations of the Factor IX can increase its susceptibility to the warfarin and its levels can fall to 1-3% while the other coagulation factors have only fallen to 30-40% levels. Such type of patients may bleed and this kind occurrence is rare (<1.5% of population).

Mutation of the gene coding for the cytochrome P450 (2C9) enzyme can affect the metabolism of the warfarin. The two forms (R and S forms) are metabolized through different pathways. The dose-response curve of the warfarin is dependent on the genetic and environmental factors. Drugs, dietary factors and diseases can influence the dose-response curve of warfarin. The anticoagulant response to warfarin is also dependent on laboratory testing, patient compliance and communication between the patient and physician. Drug to drug interaction can affect the oxidative metabolism of the S-isomer and R-isomer of warfarin. S-isomer of Warfarin is 5 times more potent than the R-isomer of warfarin. Rifampicin, barbiturates and carbamazepine increase the metabolic clearance of warfarin and so anticoagulant effect is reduced. Fluctuating levels of dietary vitamin K can overcome the vitamin K antagonist affects. Phylloquinone in the plant materials can act through warfarin insensitive reductase system and decrease the anticoagulant affect. This has been noted in the people taking weight reduction diets rich in green vegetables and vitamin K rich foods. Sick patients with hepatic dysfunction, receiving antibiotics and on IV fluids are likely to potentiate the affects of vitamin K antagonists. Aspirin and non-steroidal anti-inflammatory drugs in association with warfarin can produce gastric erosions and upper GI bleeding. If high intensity anticoagulation (INR 3.0 to 4.5) is needed then it is better to avoid the aspirin in such patients to avoid the risk of the bleeding. In our experience we feel that it is better to check the patient's INR more frequently when we are concerned about the drug or dietary interactions with warfarin.

Antithrombotic Properties of Warfarin

The antithrombotic effects of warfarin result as a consequence of reduction of Factor II, VII, IX and X. All these four factors are dependent on the Vitamin K. The anticoagulant and antithrombotic affects of warfarin are dissociated during induction period and appear at different time periods. The anticoagulant affect was noticed after 2 days of treatment and antithrombotic affects required 6 days of treatment. This finding was noted by Wessler and Gitel (1984) using the stasis model of thrombosis in rabbits. The coagulation Factors VII, IX have half-lives between 6-24 hours. But the half life of Factor II is about 96 hours. The antithrombotic effect of warfarin is due to the ability to lower the Prothrombin levels. This is the basis for the overlapping the heparin with the warfarin that is until the PT, INR has been prolonged in to the therapeutic range for at least 4 days. Based on these findings it was felt that there is no need for loading dose, as the rate of reduction of Prothrombin levels is similar with either a 5mg or a 10 mg initial warfarin dose.

Monitoring of Vitamin K Antagonist Therapy

Prothrombin time (PT) test is the most common method for monitoring oral anticoagulant therapy. The Prothrombin time is dependent on the three coagulation Factors-II, VII and X. In the initial phase of anticoagulant therapy the PT prolongation is due to reduction of factor VII, but later PT prolongation is also due to reduction of Factor X and II. Prothrombin time is measured by adding calcium, thromboplastin to the citrated plasma. Phospholipid-protein extract is known as thromboplastin. Thromboplastin is derived from the lung, brain or placenta. So, these different thromboplastins vary in their responsiveness to the vitamin K antagonist's anticoagulation affects. The less responsive thromboplastin will show less prolongation of PT for given reduction in vitamin K dependent clotting factors than a regularly responsive thromboplastin. The responsiveness of available thromboplastins is measured by assessing its international sensitivity index. Depending up on the type of thromboplastin (ISI) used the PT test results were also variable.

In the past the PT test results were found to be variable from different laboratories. It was noted that in 1980 insensitive thromboplastins (ISI 1.8-2.8) were used in USA and more responsive thromboplastins (ISI 1.0-1.4) were used in Europe. The anticoagulant dosing differences occurred in different countries [9]. This led to the search for a measure which can overcome these differences. Now, International Normalized Ratio (INR) is widely adopted in the world for monitoring oral anticoagulant therapy with vitamin K antagonists.

INR is measured as follows - INR= (patient PT/mean normal PT)^{ISI} . World Health Organization has given guidelines for ISI calibration of the thromboplastin. In many labs across the world, INR is now reported and it is more reliable than unconverted PT ratio.

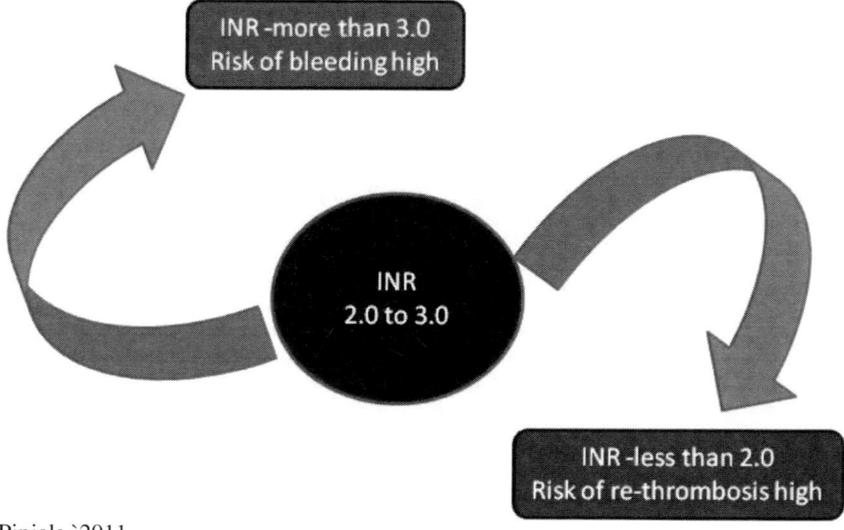

Pinjala `2011.

Figure 3. Monitoring(INR) the intensity of vitamin K antagonist in DVT patients.

What Is the Optimal Therapeutic Range of INR?

The optimal therapeutic range for the oral anticoagulant therapy was reviewed by the American college of chest physicians, National Heart Lung and Blood Institute in 1986, 1989, 1992, 1995 and 1998. INR of 2.0 to 3.0 is recommended as the therapeutic range for most conditions requiring anticoagulation. It was observed that patients with antiphospholipid antibody syndrome would require a higher targeted INR than 2.0 to 3.0.

The dose of vitamin K required to reach this therapeutic level of INR is variable in the individuals and some times in the same individual at a different times. The dietary changes, concomitant medications can increase or decrease the warfarin resistance or sensitivity of a person and affect dose requirements of the vitamin K antagonists. In clinical practice it is so important to keep track of the dietary habits of patients to understand the changes in the dose requirement. In our clinics we are often encouraging the DVT patients to get the INR test once in a week initially to remain in the therapeutic range of INR.

This helped us to maintain the TTR (Time in Therapeutic Range) 60% and above.

After 3 months of stable anticoagulation we would increase the intervals between the INR testing. If the INR values are falling below 2.0 or increasing above 3.0, then we spend more time with the patients and take detailed history and do the necessary counseling to make them understand the importance of INR and time in therapeutic range. (see Figure 3)

Duration of Vitamin K Antagonist Therapy in DVT Patients

The optimal duration of treatment with oral anticoagulants in deep vein thrombosis patients reflects a balance between the risk of recurrence when treatment is stopped and the risk of bleeding with continuation of anticoagulation therapy. If we can assess the risk of recurrence of thrombosis after stopping anticoagulation and the risk of bleeding with continuation anticoagulation, we can determine the duration of the anticoagulation therapy for the patients in our clinical practice.

Venous thrombosis is a chronic disease and recurrent events are fatal in approximately 5% to 9% of patients. [10] Predicting the likelihood of recurrence in an individual patient is of utmost importance because most recurrences can be prevented by antithrombotic therapy. The presence or absence of certain clinical and laboratory patient characteristics determines a low or high recurrence risk. The risk is low among patients with venous thromboembolism (VTE) provoked by surgery, trauma, immobilization, pregnancy or female hormone intake, whereas it is higher among those with unprovoked thrombosis. [11]

Patients who have thrombosis in the absence of known risk factors or in association with persistent risk factors (cancer and thrombophilia) are at greater risk of recurrence than the other patients with known risk factors which are time-limited and reversible. Stratification of patients with unprovoked VTE according to their recurrence risk can be achieved on the basis of clinical risk factors including patient's sex, co-morbidities, overweight or by measuring laboratory markers of thrombophilia such as factor V Leiden, the prothrombin gene mutation, natural coagulation inhibitor deficiencies, elevated coagulation factors and antiphospholipid antibodies.[12] A novel approach to assess the recurrence risk is the use of global coagulation markers, including D-dimer or in vitro thrombin generation [13, 14, 15, 16, 17].

Despite substantial progress in identifying the determinants of recurrence risk, its prediction in an individual patient is often not feasible in routine care. VTE is a disease with many causes, and the combined effect of clinical and laboratory characteristics on the risk of recurrence are unknown. The determination of some laboratory risk factors is costly, lacks standardization, or it is too elaborate for routine purposes.

Optimal duration of anticoagulation therefore should be individualized. The most important factor in assessing the risk of recurrent VTE is the relationship of the initial episode of thrombosis to risk factors. When a major reversible risk factor such as surgery can be identified as the sole explanation for VTE, then the risk of recurrence is relatively low (ie, 3% in the first year). In contrast, the risk is high (10% in the first year) in patients with unprovoked ("idiopathic") VTE and in those with persistent, irreversible, or other risk factors.

Patients in whom thrombosis was provoked by a reversible risk factor, such as leg trauma, estrogen therapy, or prolonged air travel, have an intermediate risk for recurrent VTE after stopping anticoagulant therapy (5% in the first year). Hereditary and acquired thrombophilic states associated with VTE are heterogeneous, both in terms of the frequency with which they occur in the normal population and in the strength of their association with thrombosis. Similarly the Antiphospholipid antibodies are associated with a 2-fold or greater risk of recurrent thrombosis after stopping anticoagulant therapy. One study also found that after a first episode of VTE, an anticardiolipin antibody was associated with a higher mortality during long-term follow-up because of an excess of venous and arterial thrombotic events. Continuing anticoagulant therapy appeared to reduce this risk. [18] Factor V Leiden and G20210A Prothrombin gene mutations can increase the risk of recurrent thrombosis. But, individuals with heterozygous forms of either the factor V Leiden or the G20210A prothrombin gene mutation do not appear to have a clinically important risk for recurrent VTE. Patients heterozygous for both of these mutations or homozygous for the factor V Leiden mutation appear to be at increased risk of recurrent VTE.

The deficiency of protein C, protein S and antithrombin III are associated with thrombosis risk. But there is little prospective information on the risk of recurrent VTE in patients with antithrombin III, protein C, or protein S deficiency. In patients with 1 of these abnormalities or a lupus anticoagulant, a prospective study identified a hazard ratio of 1.4 for recurrent VTE. [19] In another study, relative risks for recurrent VTE were 1.0 for protein S, 1.8 for protein C, and 2.6 for antithrombin III deficiency.[20] In a retrospective family cohort study, the presence of 1 of these abnormalities was associated with a 10% cumulative frequency of recurrent VTE in the first year after diagnosis and a 23% frequency by 5 years. [21]

Therefore, although there is uncertainty, these abnormalities do not appear to be clinically important risk factors for recurrent VTE. Elevated Factor VIII levels (>200 IU/dL) are known to be associated with recurrent thrombosis, surprisingly in clinical practice it is still not common to check for this abnormality routinely. Hyperhomocystinemia can be congenital or acquired and it is known to increase the risk of recurrent thrombosis 2.7 folds. However lowering of the homocysteine did not convincingly reduce the risk of recurrent thrombosis in the trials.

Cancer patients are higher risk of thrombosis and recurrent thrombosis. The patients with metastasis have 3 folds greater risk of recurrent thrombosis than those with localized tumors. If anticoagulation is stopped in cancer patients the risk recurrent thrombosis in the first year can be as high as 10% to 20%. It is more likely in those with poor mobility, progressive cancer, metastatic cancer and receiving chemotherapy. If the initial venous thrombosis in cancer patients was precipitated by surgery or chemotherapy then probably the risk of recurrent venous thrombosis may be less.

Are There Differences in Recurrence of Thrombosis in Deep Vein Thrombosis and Pulmonary Embolism Patients?

Patients who developed pulmonary thromboembolism and those with only proximal deep vein thrombosis are known to have similar risk of recurrent thrombosis. [22] Patients who had initially pulmonary embolism are more likely (>60%) to develop a recurrent episodes in the form of pulmonary embolism only.

When the initial episode was deep vein thrombosis, the recurrence in them is only 20% in the form of pulmonary embolism and the rest would be only deep vein thrombosis. That means the risk of recurrent pulmonary embolism is 3 folds higher in the pulmonary embolism patients than in the deep vein thrombosis patients. Case fatality rates for late recurrent thrombosis in pulmonary embolism and deep vein thrombosis are 10% and 5%. Though the incidence of recurrent thrombosis is same in pulmonary embolism patients and deep vein thrombosis patients, the case fatality rates are two fold higher in recurrent pulmonary embolism patients. [23] Patients with chronic pulmonary hypertension due to venous thromboembolism are usually given anticoagulation indefinitely if there is no contraindication to prevent further episodes of recurrent thrombosis which can be fatal.

Can Residual Deep Vein Thrombosis after Initial Therapies Determine the Risk of Recurrent Deep Vein Thrombosis to Consider Long-Term Anticoagulation?

Treatment of deep venous thrombosis with anticoagulants will result in recanalization of the thrombus or complete resolution of thrombus. The degree of recanalization is variable and dependent on many factors and time. Thrombin bound to the thrombus is difficult to be neutralized during the treatment with anticoagulants. If there is large amount of residual thrombus burden then there is a possibility of increased incidence of recurrence of thrombosis.

It was observed that if there is residual proximal deep vein thrombosis after 3 months of initial anticoagulation therapy there is a 3-fold increased risk of recurrent thrombosis. In patients with PE and concomitant DVT, 3 months after initial anticoagulation therapy the risk of recurrent thrombosis was found to be increased by 1.4-fold. Though the recurrent thrombosis in known to occur in those with residual thrombosis, it is probably not due to the obstruction to the venous flow. The equal distribution of the recurrent DVT in the initially affected and unaffected legs suggests that the cause for recurrence could be due to some factors other than obstruction to the venous flows. Inferior vena cava filters doubled the risk of recurrent DVT over 2 years but there has been no increase in the pulmonary embolism. [24] So, patients with Inferior vena cava filters will require long term anticoagulation with vitamin K antagonists to prevent recurrent thrombosis.

The Bleeding Risk in DVT Patients Receiving Vitamin K Antagonists – Anticoagulation over a Long Period of Time

We would generally give anticoagulation for 3 to 6 months after an attack of deep vein thrombosis. If the anticoagulation with vitamin K antagonists is continued after that period to maintain the INR between 2.0 to 3.0, it can increase the risk of bleeding. The average rate of major bleeding in such situations can be 2% per year in patients with VTE. Approximately 10% of these major bleeds occurring in patients taking long term oral anticoagulation can be fatal [25] Major hemorrhage occurs with a rate of 2.4% to 8% per patient-year.

Vitamin K antagonists increase the risk of intracranial hemorrhage (ICH) 7- to 10-fold, to a rate of nearly 1% per patient-year. ICH has an estimated 60% mortality rate. The risk of bleeding is variable in individual patients. The factors that are known to influence the risk of bleeding are Age, history of GI bleeding, stroke, chronic renal disease, metastatic malignancy, alcohol-related disease or diabetes and concomitant medication with antiplatelet drugs. In the recent past there has been a search for the genetic predisposition for the bleeding risk in patients receiving the anticoagulation therapy. Hereditary factors such as polymorphisms of the cytochrome P450 system may precipitate bleeding in patients receiving the vitamin K antagonists. This type of bleeding is likely to happen during initial phase of anticoagulation as the underlying problem is genetic in nature.

Skin Necrosis due to Vitamin K Antagonist Therapy

Warfarin-induced skin necrosis is rare and it is a serious complication of oral anticoagulant therapy. It has a prevalence of 0.01-0.1%. This was first recognized in 1943. Warfarin-induced skin necrosis usually occurs in middle-aged, peri-menopausal and obese women who are being treated with warfarin for thromboembolic disease. It develops within 1-10 days of initiating warfarin therapy. The majority of cases appear between day 3 and 6 of therapy. Late onset warfarin-induced skin necrosis occurs rarely from 15 days up to 15 years after onset of therapy. Skin necrosis usually appears in microcirculation-rich areas. In women, breast, buttocks and thighs are the most common sites; in men, the penile skin may be affected. In our unit we have also seen involvement of trunk, extremities. Few patients are also seen face involvement also. Pathological changes include extensive thrombosis with microvascular injury and fibrin deposits in the postcapillary venules and small veins. There is no vascular or perivascular inflammation.

The arteriolar thrombosis is absent and it is a distinctive feature. Clinically they present with paresthesia, sensation of pressure with an erythematous flush, and /or skin discomfort. The lesions are demarcated, painful, and initially hemorrhagic. Hemorrhagic bullae and full-thickness skin necrosis with eschar formation are seen in the late stages.

They can spontaneously heal after discontinuation of warfarin. Recurrence of skin necrosis in the absence of further anticoagulation therapy has been reported. Whether the condition reappears or not is unpredictable after restarting the drug. The precise cause of the disease is unclear. Protein C deficiency, protein S deficiency, factor VII deficiency, hypersensitivity, direct toxic effect of warfarin, and other mechanisms have all been proposed. Among these, protein C deficiency is a widely accepted major risk factor. This phenomenon may be explained by the rapid drop in factor VII and protein C levels (as they have a half-life of only 5 hours) following the initiation of warfarin. This transiently procoagulant nature further exaggerated in protein C deficiency, leading to a relative hypercoagulable state which can lead to thrombotic occlusion of the microvasculature. In addition to protein C deficiency, other Hypercoagulable conditions, such as protein S deficiency, resistance to activated protein C, antithrombin III deficiency and lupus anticoagulants have been associated with warfarin-induced skin necrosis.

Heparin is also known to cause skin necrosis which can be clinically indistinguishable from warfarin-induced skin necrosis. The heparin-induced version is more commonly seen in abdominal wall, extremities and nose. Heparin induced necrosis appears between 5- 10 days after onset of therapy. The associated morbidity is high with skin necrosis. More than 50% of the patients would require surgical intervention with wide local debridement, skin grafting or even amputation. Failure of early diagnosis and treatment may result in death.

Duration of Anticoagulant Therapy (Figure 4 below)

One would like to shorten the duration of vitamin K antagonist therapy as they are going to be less expensive. But the studies have shown that if we follow the short term anticoagulation with vitamin K antagonists the risk of recurrent thrombosis is doubled in the heterogeneous group of patients.

Major bleeding was uncommon (2.7% per year) during the period of long term anticoagulation. Some think that calf vein thrombosis with a transient risk factor can be safely treated with 6 weeks of anticoagulation only. But this is not recommended for the proximal DVT or PE as there is doubling of the VTE risk associated with the short term anticoagulation.

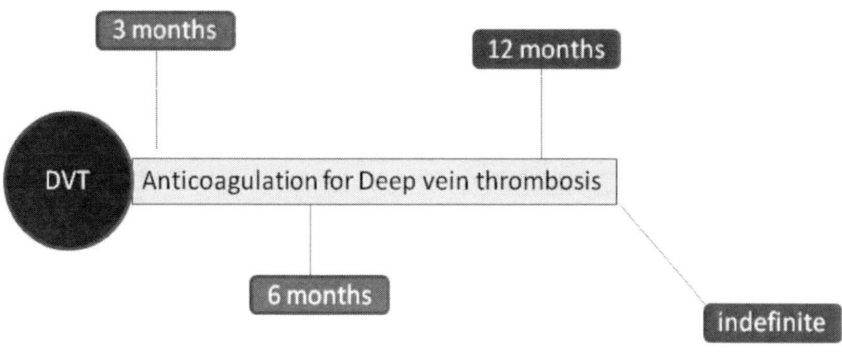

Pinjala `2011.

Figure 4.

In another study, Pinede et al 3 months of anticoagulation was compared with 6 months of anticoagulation and there was no difference between the two groups at the end of 15 months. [26] Interestingly, Agnelli et al compared the 3 months anticoagulation with one year anticoagulation and found out that the recurrent VTE was less in those who received anticoagulation for one year (3% vs. 8.3%). But this benefit did not sustain 2 year after stopping the anticoagulation. We choose the duration of anticoagulation which can balance reduction of recurrent thrombosis against the bleeding.[27] Case fatality rates are higher after PE than after DVT due to recurrent VTE though the risk of major bleeding may be similar. Studies have shown that 90% of recurrent thrombotic attacks can be prevented by anticoagulation with an annual risk of 2% major bleeding, that means the long term anticoagulation is justified if the VTE risk exceeds 1.5% after PE and 3% after DVT to offset a fatal bleeding. [28]

Time in Therapeutic Range (TTR)

When vitamin K antagonists are given to the patients for long periods to prevent recurrent thrombosis, it is important know for how much amount of time the patients are remaining in the therapeutic range of INR. Some time when patients forget to take the tablets, dietary changes or drug interactions there can be variation in the INR. We need a good measure to know for how much time in between the two clinic visits the patient is remaining in the therapeutic range.

The doses can be adjusted more frequently if needed. It was found that in majority of studies people were in maintaining a TTR 50-60%. It is difficult to maintain the TTR values above the 60%.

There three types of calculations to measure the TTR. At the National Conference on Anticoagulation Therapy on 22nd May 2007, a presentation was given by Scott Kaatz, MD, regarding the different metrics for determining therapeutic time in range.

Percent of Visits in Range (Traditional Method)

This looks at how many visits had INR results in range, and divides by the total number of visits. If the patient has had 8 visits, and 6 had readings within their therapeutic range, then the patient is considered in range 75% of the time.

Percent of Visits in Range on Given Date (Cross Section Method)

This method takes a specific date in time, and all patients are evaluated on the last reading prior to that date to see if they were within range. The number of patients in range (on their last reading) is taken as a percentage of the total active patients on that date.

Percent of Days in Range (Rosendaal Method)

This is the most complex of the calculations, as it looks at the amount of time between visits to determine how long the patient might have been within their therapeutic range. If a patient has a therapeutic range of 2.0-3.0, and on May 1st tested at 2.5, then tested 3.5 on May 31st, then we can determine how many days were in range. Since there were 30 days between tests, you assume that the patient slowly moved from 2.5 to 3.5 over those 30 days, so around May 15th, the patient was probably over 3.0, and therefore was out of range. Therefore, we estimate that 15 days were in range, and 15 days were out of range (within the 30 day time period), which means the patient is within range 50% of the time. Madeleine et al group from Canada showed that in long-term care residents, warfarin control was suboptimal. Both prescriber and co-prescription of interacting medications were associated with poorer INR control. Future studies should seek strategies to improve prescriber skill and decrease use of interacting medications. Their study is the first to assess TTR in long term care residents on warfarin in Canada. They found that the quality of anticoagulant care was sub-optimal; overall, INR was in the therapeutic range 54% of the time and was sub therapeutic 35% of the time. The majority of residents received at least one warfarin-interacting drug. Eighty-two percent of times an interacting drug was started, INR testing occurred within one week, which compares favorably to monitoring in a study in outpatients (INR testing within 14 days, 77% of the time). [29] Despite monitoring, TTR was lower in residents receiving warfarin-interacting medications. The quality of anticoagulation also varied significantly between physicians (TTR 45.9 to 63.3%). The overall TTR result they obtained was comparable with that reported in three previous studies (TTR range 40 to 51%). However, the values compare unfavourably with an average TTR of 61% in studies in outpatients receiving warfarin. [30]

Management of Excessive Anticoagulant Affect with Elevated INR with or without Bleeding While Receiving Vitamin K Antagonists

It is common to see the unexpectedly elevated INR values in our clinical practice. In the absence of bleeding, such values may be treated with either simple warfarin withdrawal in general or the administration of low doses of oral vitamin K in some countries. Oral vitamin K will more rapidly return the INR to the therapeutic reference interval, but its impact on bleeding is still unknown. If the INR is more than 10, most of us recommend the administration of vitamin K and, in the case of active bleeding, we recommend administration of coagulation factors either in the form of fresh frozen plasma (FFP) or prothrombin complex concentrates (PCC). Coagulation factor replacement is required to urgently correct the INR and along with vitamin K to antagonize the effect of warfarin. Vitamin K prevents the "rebound" anticoagulation when the transfused coagulation factors are consumed. An elevated INR independently predicts major bleeding. The risk of bleeding approximately doubles for each single point of increase in the INR above 3.0. [31, 32] Major hemorrhage occurs with a rate of 2.4% to 8% per patient-year. Vitamin K anatgonists increase the risk of intracranial hemorrhage (ICH) 7- to 10-fold, to a rate of nearly 1% per patient-year. ICH has an estimated 60% mortality rate. [25, 33, 34]

Management of Non-bleeding Patient with High INR Values

Conservative treatment of non-bleeding over-anticoagulated patients entails simply withholding VKA and allowing the INR to fall into the therapeutic range. This is the most widely used approach to the treatment of patients with warfarin-associated coagulopathy. The recommendation to simply withhold VKA and allow the INR to fall into the desired range is supported by two case series in which a total of 352 INR values above 6.0 occurred in 299 patients. Only 2 patients (0.6%) suffered haemorrhage when treated with simple temporary withdrawal of VKA. [35, 36]

In a more recent and larger series Garcia et al evaluated the 30-day incidence of major bleeding in patients with INR above 5 this risk was low (1.3%). Vitamin K use in this study was infrequent. When patients with INR value above 9 were evaluated separately the 30-day risk of major bleeding was high (9.6%), calling into question the safety of this approach in patients with higher INR values. Three studies have compared intravenous vitamin K in differing doses for the treatment of VKA-associated coagulopathy. These studies concluded that a 0.5 mg intravenous dose was optimal if the goal of therapy was to return the INR to the usual therapeutic range. Although anaphylactoid reactions have been described with the intravenous vitamin K1 most such cases occurred with large doses of vitamin K, administered rapidly and with little dilution. The best estimate of the frequency of this complication is about 3 per 10, 000 doses administered; it may be more likely if formulations containing polyethoxylated castor oil are used to maintain the vitamin K in solution. Modern formulations of vitamin K for intravenous injection utilize solubilizers that appear to be associated with a lower risk of anaphylaxis.

Management of Patients Who Require Urgent Reversal of Anticoagulation

Patients who are bleeding while receiving VKAs or those who are in need of immediate surgery require urgent reversal of anticoagulation. Management of these patients must be individualized. The severity and location of the hemorrhage and the INR level when bleeding determine the management. Major hemorrhage occurs with a rate of 2.4% to 8% per patient-year. Vitamin K Antagonists increase the risk of intracranial hemorrhage (ICH) 7- to 10-fold, to a rate of nearly 1% per patient-year. ICH has an estimated 60% mortality rate.

VKA therapy should be withheld in all patients with major bleeding during VKA therapy. Patients should receive intravenous vitamin K and coagulation factor replacement. Intravenously administered vitamin K works more rapidly than either oral or subcutaneous vitamin K. The INR starts showing correction within 2 hours, and it can come to normal range within 24 hours if hepatic function is normal with a sufficient dose of vitamin K is given. The low-dose vitamin K (0.5 to 1 mg) without coagulation factor replacement is inappropriate when rapid correction is needed. FFP is widely available in our blood banks and it provides rapid but partial reversal of coagulopathy through replacement of coagulation factors II, VII, IX, and X.

In many hospitals FFP remains the most widely used coagulation factor replacement product for urgent reversal of VKA. The usual dose of plasma is 15 mL/kg, although the optimal dose has not been established. A lower dose (5 to 8 mL/kg) may be appropriate when urgent reversal of a therapeutic (rather than supra therapeutic) INR is required. [37, 38, 39] Prothrombin complex concentrates (PCCs) provide a rapid and effective method for replacing deficient clotting factors and correcting INR. It may be preferable to plasma if it is readily available. PCCs are intermediate-purity pooled plasma products containing factors II, IX, and X with variable amounts of FVII and natural anticoagulant proteins C and S. They were previously used in the treatment of hemophilia B prior to the availability of high-purity plasma-derived and recombinant FIX concentrates.

In the first controlled trial, Taberner et al randomized 18 overanticoagulated patients to receive PCC or intravenous vitamin K. [40]. Patients randomized to PCC had a more rapid INR correction compared to patients randomized to vitamin K. Several additional (but small) prospective studies have shown that PCC is effective in reducing INR and achieving rapid hemostasis in patients with major bleeding or who required urgent surgery. PCCs are likely to produce more rapid and complete INR reversal compared with FFP. In a study conducted on 41 patients who were bleeding because of warfarin over dosage or who required urgent reversal of warfarin therapy, Makris et al compared the efficacy of PCC (25-50 U/kg) and FFP for rapidly reducing INR. Complete correction of the INR occurred within 15 minutes in 28 of 29 patients treated with PCC versus none of 12 patients treated with FFP.[41] However, whether PCC improves clinical outcome when compared with FFP is unknown. As with other coagulation factor concentrates there remains a risk of transfusion-transmitted infection; however, this risk is significantly reduced by procedures such as solvent/detergent-treatment and nanofiltration. The optimal dose of PCC is not established, and some experts suggest that should be individualized according to initial INR, target INR and body weight. Furthermore, available data do not allow a direct comparison among different PCCs. In a randomized trial, van Aart et al showed that the number of patients reaching the target-INR 15 minutes after the dosage of PCC was significantly higher in the group treated with an "individualized" dosage, compared to the group treated with a standard dose (89% vs 43%; $P < .001$). In another recent study, Yasaka et al found that 500 IU of the PCCs were sufficient for rapid correction of INR values below 5.0 but that they were inadequate in patients with INR values of 5.0 or more in patients with major hemorrhagic complications of anticoagulant treatment or who required invasive procedures. [42]

Fear of thrombotic complications has limited the use of PCCs even in patients presenting with life-threatening haemorrhage. However, in a systematic review including 14 studies for a total of 460 patients, there were only 7 thrombotic complications (3 strokes, 2 myocardial infarctions and 2 deep vein thromboses).[43] Recombinant FVIIa (rFVIIa) has been used in patients with acute intra cerebral haemorrhage who were not receiving anticoagulant therapy. Although earlier results were promising, a larger randomized trial failed to confirm rFVIIa reduced mortality. rVIIa has also been used for correction of warfarin associated coagulopathy; it effectively corrected the INR in healthy human volunteers receiving acenocoumarol [44] and it appears to rapidly correct the INR in excessively anticoagulated patients and in patients presenting with central nervous system bleeding emergencies. [45] However, rVIIa causes thrombosis and there are few data to support its clinical efficacy; as a result its routine use should be avoided until better quality evidence supporting its effectiveness becomes available. If rVIIa is used it is important to remember to administer vitamin K and to monitor closely for recurrent coagulopathy as it has a half-life of less than 60 minutes.

Can We Replace Vitamin K Antagonists with Unfractionated Heparin, LMWH and Oral Direct Thrombin Inhibitors?

Various subcutaneous heparin regimens have been used instead of Vitamin K antagonists to treat VTE for 3 or 6 months. Of these studies, the 13 most recent compared widely differing LMWH regimens with VK antagonists (INR 2.0 to 3.0) or, in 1 small study, unfractionated heparin. Three months of low-dose unfractionated heparin (5000 U twice daily) was inadequate treatment for proximal DVT. Three or 6 months of unfractionated heparin or LMWH, in doses that varied from one third to full therapeutic doses were effective.

A meta-analysis of 7 of these studies (total of 1379 patients) found 3 months of LMWH therapy associated with less recurrent VTE (odds ratio 0.7; 95% CI, 0.4 to 1.1) and less major bleeding (odds ratio 0.4; 95% CI, 0.2 to 1.1) than treatment with a VK antagonist for 3 months. Compared with VK antagonists, between-study differences in mean daily dose of LMWH had little effect on efficacy but did influence bleeding (odds ratio of 0.2 with 4000 IU/d to 0.7 with 12 000 IU/d for major bleeding relative to the VK antagonist groups). Two studies not included in this analysis suggest that prolonged treatment with LMWH is preferable to VK antagonists in patients with active cancer. In the larger of these 2 studies (700 patients), daily injections of LMWH (dalteparin 200 IU/kg for the first month and then 150 IU/kg for 5 months) was associated with half the frequency of recurrent VTE during 6 months of treatment (9% versus 17% with VK antagonists) with no significant increase in major bleeding (6% versus 4%). In the future oral direct thrombin inhibitors may be showing improvements and clinical benefits, we need to compare them with warfarin therapies. However the cost of the new drugs may be more than warfarin and it will take some more time for the change over to the newer drugs even if the initial results are looking better. Unitl then Vitamin K antagonists are going to be used optimally with adequate monitoring.

References

[1]   Kyrle PA, Eichinger S. Deep vein thrombosis. *Lancet.* 2005; 465: 1163-74.

[2]   Linkins LA, Choi PT, Douketis JD. Clinical impact of bleeding in patients taking oral anticoagulant therapy for venous thromboembolism: a meta-analysis. *Ann. Intern. Med.* 2003; 139: 893-900.

[3]   Barritt DW, Jordan SC. Anticoagulant drugs in the treatment of pulmonary embolism. A controlled trial. *Lancet.* 1960; 1 (7138): 1309-12.

[4]   Brandjes DP, Heijboer H, Buller HR, et al. Acenocoumarol and heparin compared with acenocoumarol alone in the initial treatment of proximal-vein thrombosis. *N. Engl. J. Med.* 1992; 327 (21): 1485-9.

[5]   Hull R, Delmore T, Genton E, et al. Warfarin sodium versus low-dose heparin in the long-term treatment of venous thrombosis. *N. Engl. J. Med.* 1979; 301 (16): 855-8.

[6]   Paterson JM et al. Clinical consequences of generic warfarin substitution: an ecological study. *JAMA.* 2006; 296 (16): 1969-72.

[7]   Salzman EW, Davies GC. Prophylaxis of venous thromboembolism: analysis of cost effectiveness. *Ann. Surg.* 1980; 191 (2): 207-18.

[8]   Paiement GD, Bell D, Wessinger SJ, Harris WH. New advances in the prevention, diagnosis, and cost effectiveness of venous thromboembolic disease in patients with total hip replacement. In Brand RD (ed) the Hip. St Louis: CB Mosby, 1987, pp94-199.

[9]   Poller L, Taberner DA. Dosage and control of oral anticoagulants: an international collaborative survey. *Br. J. Haemotol.* 1982; 51 (3): 479-85.

[10]   Douketis JD, Gu CS, Schuman S, Ghirarduzzi A. The risk for fatal pulmonary embolism after discontinuing anticoagulant therapy for venous thromboembolism. *Ann. Intern. Med.* 2007; 147 (11): 766-74.

[11]   Kearon C, Kahn SR, Agnelli G, Goldhaber SZ, Raskob G, Comerota AJ. Antithrombotic Therapy for Venous Thromboembolic Disease: ACCP Evidence- Based Clinical Practice Guidelines (8th Edition). *Chest.* 2008; 133(6 Suppl): 454S-545S.

[12]   Zhu T, Martinez I, Emmerich J. Venous thromboembolism: risk factors for recurrence. *Arterioscler. Thromb. Vasc. Biol.* 2009; 29 (3): 298-310.

[13]   Verhovsek M, Douketis JD, Yi Q, Shrivastava S, Tait RC. Systematic review: D-dimer to predict recurrent disease after stopping anticoagulant therapy for unprovoked venous thromboembolism. *Ann. Intern. Med.* 2008; 149 (7): 481-90, W94.

[14]   Hron G, Kollars M, Binder BR, Eichinger S, Kyrle PA. Identification of patients at low risk for recurrent venous thromboembolism by measuring thrombin generation. *JAMA.* 2006; 296 (4): 397-402.

[15]   Eichinger S, Hron G, Kollars M, Kyrle PA. Prediction of recurrent venous thromboembolism by endogenous thrombin potential and D-dimer. *Clin. Chem.* 2008; 54 (12): 2042-8.

[16]   Tripodi A, Legnani C, Chantarangkul V, Cosmi B. High thrombin generation measured in the presence of thrombomodulin is associated with an increased risk of recurrent venous thromboembolism. *J. Thromb. Haemost.* 2008; 6 (8): 1327-33.

[17]   Besser M, Baglin C, Luddington R, van Hylckama Vlieg A. High rate of unprovoked recurrent venous thrombosis is associated with high thrombin-generating potential in a prospective cohort study. *J. Thromb. Haemost.* 2008; 6 (10): 1720-5.

[18]   Schulman S, Svenungsson E, Granqvist S. Anticardiolipin antibodies predict early recurrence of thromboembolism and death among patients with venous thromboembolism following anticoagulant therapy. Duration of Anticoagulation Study Group. *Am. J. Med.* 1998; 104 (4): 332-8.

[19] Prandoni P, Lensing AWA, Cogo A, et al. The long-term clinical course of acute deep venous thrombosis. *Ann. Intern. Med.* 1996; 125 (1): 1-7125.

[20] Baglin T, Luddington R, Brown K, et al. Incidence of recurrent venous thromboembolism in relation to clinical and thrombophilic risk factors: prospective cohort study. *Lancet.* 2003; 362 (9383): 523-6.

[21] Van den Belt AG, Sanson BJ, Simioni P, et al. Recurrence of venous thromboembolism in patients with familial thrombophilia. *Arch. Intern. Med.* 1997; 157 (19): 2227-32.

[22] Heit JA, Mohr DN, Silverstein MD, et al. Predictors of recurrence after deep vein thrombosis and pulmonary embolism: a population-based cohort study. *Arch. Intern. Med.* 2000; 160 (6): 761-8.

[23] Douketis JD, Kearon C, Bates S, et al. Risk of fatal pulmonary embolism in patients with treated venous thromboembolism. *JAMA.* 1998; 279(6): 458-62.

[24] Decousus H, Leizorovicz A, Parent F, et al. A clinical trial of vena caval filters in the prevention of pulmonary embolism in patients with proximal deep-vein thrombosis. Prévention du Risque d'Embolie Pulmonaire par Interruption Cave Study Group. *N. Engl. J. Med.* 1998; 338(7): 409-15.

[25] Linkins L, Choi PT, Douketis JD. Clinical impact of bleeding in patients taking oral anticoagulant therapy for venous thromboembolism: a meta-analysis. *Ann. Intern. Med.* 2003; 139 (11): 893-900.

[26] Pinede L, Ninet J, Duhaut P, et al. Comparison of 3 and 6 months of oral anticoagulant therapy after a first episode of proximal deep vein thrombosis or pulmonary embolism and comparison of 6 and 12 weeks of therapy after isolated calf deep vein thrombosis. *Circulation.* 200; 103 (20): 2453-60.

[27] Agnelli G, Prandoni P, Santamaria MG, et al. Three months versus one year of oral anticoagulant therapy for idiopathic deep venous thrombosis. Warfarin Optimal Duration Italian Trial Investigators. *N. Engl. J. Med.* 2001; 345 (3): 165-9.

[28] Kearon C, Gent M, Hirsh J, et al. A comparison of three months of anticoagulation with extended anticoagulation for a first episode of idiopathic venous thromboembolism. *N. Engl. J. Med.* 1999; 340 (12): 901-7.

[29] Raebel MA, Witt DM, Carroll NM, Magid DJ. Warfarin monitoring in ambulatory older individuals receiving antimicrobial therapy. *Pharmacotherapy* 2005; 25 (8): 1055-6.

[30] Reynolds MW, Fahrbach K, Hauch O, Wygant G, Estok R, Cella C. Warfarin anticoagulation and outcomes in patients with atrial fibrillation: a systematic review and metaanalysis. *Chest.* 2004; 126 (6): 1938-45.

[31] Hylek EM, Chang YC, Skates SJ, Hughes RA, Singer DE. Prospective study of the outcomes of ambulatory patients with excessive warfarin anticoagulation. *Arch. Intern. Med.* 2000; 160 (11): 1612-7.

[32] Landefeld CS, Rosenblatt MW, Goldman L. Bleeding in outpatients treated with warfarin: relation to the prothrombin time and important remediable lesions. *Am. J. Med.* 1989; 87 (2): 153-9.

[33] Fitzmaurice DA, Blann AD, Lip GY. Bleeding risks of antithrombotic therapy. *Br. Med. J.* 2002; 325(7368): 828-31.

[34] Hart RG, Boop BS, Anderson DC. Oral anticoagulants and intracranial hemorrhage. Facts and hypotheses. *Stroke.* 1995; 26 (8): 1471-7.

[35] Glover JJ, Morrill GB. Conservative treatment of overanticoagulated patients. *Chest.* 1995; 108 (4): 987-90.

[36] Lousberg TR, Witt DM, Beall DG, Carter BL, Malone DC. Evaluation of excessive anticoagulation in a group model health maintenance organization. *Arch. Intern. Med.* 1998; 158 (5): 528-34.

[37] Baglin T. Management of warfarin (coumarin) overdose. *Blood Rev.* 1998; 12 (2): 91-8.

[38] Contreras M, Ala FA, Greaves M, et al. Guidelines for the use of fresh frozen plasma. British Committee for Standards in Haematology, Working Party of the Blood Transfusion Task Force. *Transfus. Med.* 1992; 2 (1): 57-63.

[39] Guidelines for red blood cell and plasma transfusion for adults and children. Report of the Expert Working Group. *CMAJ.* 1997; 156 (11): S1-S24.

[40] Taberner DA, Thomson JM, Poller L. Comparison of prothrombin complex concentrate and vitamin K1 in oral anticoagulant reversal. *Br. Med. J.* 1976; 2 (6027): 83-5.

[41] Makris M, Greaves M, Phillips WS, Kitchen S. *Thromb. Haemost.* 77, 477 (1997).

[42] Yasaka M, Sakata T, Naritomi H, Minematsu K. Optimal dose of prothrombin complex concentrate for acute reversal of oral anticoagulation. *Thromb. Res.* 2005; 115 (6): 455-9.

[43] Leissinger CA, Blatt PM, Hoots WK, Ewenstein B. Role of prothrombin complex concentrates in reversing warfarin anticoagulation: a review of the literature. *Am. J. Hematol.* 2008; 83 (2): 137-43.

[44] Erhardtsen E, Nony P, Dechavanne M, Ffrench P. The effect of recombinant factor VIIa (NovoSeven) in healthy volunteers receiving acenocoumarol to an International Normalized Ratio above 2.0. *Blood Coagul. Fibrinolysis.* 1998; 9(8): 741-8.

[45] Sorensen B, Johansen P, Nielsen GL, Sorensen JC. Reversal of the International Normalized Ratio with recombinant activated factor VII in central nervous system bleeding during warfarin thromboprophylaxis: clinical and biochemical aspects. Blood Coagul. *Fibrinolysis.* 2003; 14 (5): 469-77.

In: Deep Vein Thrombosis
Editor: Takashi Yamaki

ISBN: 978-1-62257-519-0
© 2013 Nova Science Publishers, Inc.

Chapter 7

Surgical Treatment of Acute Deep Vein Thrombosis

Tomohiro Ogawa[*]
Department of Cardiovascular surgery,
Fukushima Daiichi Hospital, Japan

Abstract

The ilio-femoral venous thrombosis has higher risks of fatal pulmonary embolism, severe pain and swelling, moreover developing ischemia of the affected leg. In addition, the disabling post-thrombotic syndrome (PTS) which causes the pain, swelling, pigmentation or ulceration of legs is often found as late complications. The anticoagulant therapy is a widely accepted treatment for acute deep vein thrombosis to prevent pulmonary embolism and recurrent deep vein thrombosis with strong evidence. However, the results of anticoagulants are not always satisfied from the points of eliminating patient's complaints quickly and further prevention of PTS. Several reports show that the early removal of venous thrombus plays an important role of maintaining venous valvular competence and preventing PTS. So catheter-directed thrombolysis (CDT) and surgical thrombectomy, which can be expected, and early

[*] Correspondence to: TomohiroOgawa MD, Department of Cardiovascular surgery, Fukushima Daiichi Hospital, 16-2 Kitasawamata, Nariide, Fukushima City, Fukushima, 960-8251 Japan. Tel: +81-24-557-5111. Fax: +81-24-557-5064. E-mail: tomo-ogawa@msb.biglobe.ne.jp.

removal of venous thrombus are considered aggressive treatments of ilio-femoral venous thrombosis to relieve symptom quickly and prevent post-thrombotic syndrome more than anticoagulant therapy alone. Since the excellent thrombolytic result of CDT was reported with less invasive, venous thrombectomy is becoming an alternative method of CDT. Currently, the surgical thrombectomy tends to be indicated for mobilized patients who have acute ilio-femoral thrombus with the contraindication or failure of thrombolysis.

Thrombectomy for ilio-femoral venous thrombosis is approached from the common femoral vein using a Fogarty catheter and manual massage under general anesthesia with the protection of peri-operative pulmonary thromboembolism. The construction of temporary A-V fistula and additional endovenous procedures such as stenting for the stenotic iliac vein are recommended to maintain the patency of the ilio-femoral vein.

Previous reports show the early and late results of surgical thrombectomy with selected indications are fairly good. The surgical thrombectomy is still an option for the treatment of severe acute ilio-femoral vein thrombosis.

Introduction

The ilio-femoral venous thrombosis has higher risks of fatal pulmonary embolism, severe pain and swelling leading to compartment syndrome with phlegmasia cerulea dolens and venous gangrene. In addition, the disabling post-thrombotic syndrome (PTS) with pain, venous claudication, swelling, pigmentation or ulceration of legs. The anticoagulant therapy is a widely accepted treatment for acute deep vein thrombosis to prevent pulmonary embolism and recurrent deep vein thrombosis with strong evidence [1]. However, the results of anticoagulants are not always satisfactory from the points of eliminating patient's complaints quickly and prevention of PTS. Several reports show that early removal of venous thrombus plays an important role of maintaining venous patency and valvular competence thereby preventing PTS [2-5]. Catheter directed thrombolysis (CDT) and surgical thrombectomy are considered as aggressive treatments of ilio-femoral venous thrombosis to relieve symptoms quickly and prevent post-thrombotic syndrome more than anticoagulant therapy alone. Endovenous treatment of ilio-femoral DVT is less invasive and is therefore the first choice leaving surgical thrombectomy as an alternative [1, 6].

Indication of Surgical Thrombectomy

Currently, surgical thrombectomy is indicated for ambulatory patients who have symptoms such as severe pain, swelling or developed ischemia with a good life expectancy. The contraindication or failure of thrombolysis is one of indications of surgical thrombectomy.

The deep vein thrombus should be extended into the ilio-femoral vein and the clot age should be less than 7 days. Clot age has an influence on the thrombus removal and valve destruction, treatment of the younger clot is expected to give a better clinical outcome. Clot age is estimated from the onset of symptoms, however, clot age sometimes may be older than the time from the onset of symptoms.

Surgical Technique

Thrombectomy for ilio-femoral venous thrombosis is approached from the common femoral vein using a Fogarty catheter and manual massage under general anesthesia with the protection of peri-operative pulmonary thromboembolism using IVC occlusion balloon, temporary IVC filter and positive end expiratory pressure (PEEP) ventilation. A venotomy is placed at the common femoral vein. The venous Fogarty thormbectomy catheter is inserted into IVC and proximal thrombus in the iliac vein is removed by pulling the thrombectomy catheter with the inflated balloon. In the case that the thrombus extends to the popliteal vein or calf veins, this distal thrombus is removed by manual massage of the elevated leg. When the removal of the distal thrombus is not possible by manual massage, it can be removed by a Fogarty catheter, with a caution for injury of venous valves. As an idea for further distal thrombectomy, it is reported that a small Fogarty catheter is inserted from opened posterior tibial vein to common femoral vein as a guide for a large Fogarty catheter from the proximal side and the distal thrombus is flushed out by an infusion of saline solution from the posterior tibial vein after thrombectomy [7].

In the case of incomplete removal of femoro-popliteal thrombus due to extensive and old thrombus, Eklof has recommended the complete removal of thrombus through the deep femoral vein with smaller Fogarty catheters, because the deep femoral venous tract becomes an important collateral flow keeping the iliac vein patent. The femoral vein can then be ligated avoiding the development of deep venous reflux [8].

The clearance of thrombus or remaining stenosis and occlusion in the iliac vein should be confirmed using completion venography. In remaining occlusion or stenosis of the iliac vein after thrombectomy, stenting or balloon angioplasty is recommended (Figure 1) [9-12]. Peri-operative regional thrombolysis is also tried to combine with thrombectomy for better outcome. [13].

Also, the construction of temporary A-V fistula using the saphenous vein or prosthesis is recommended to maintain the patency of ilio-femoral vein [14].

A recent report showed that A-V fistula for maintaining the patency of the ilio-femoral vein after complete clearance of ilio-femoral vein thrombus may not be necessary [11].

Temporary A-V fistula is closed after 1 -2 months. Heparin is continued at least 5 days and oral anticoagulants continued for 6 months. The compression therapy is recommended for two years. Intermittent pneumatic compression is an alternative if the patient is not ambulating at the post-operative period (Table 1) [7, 15].

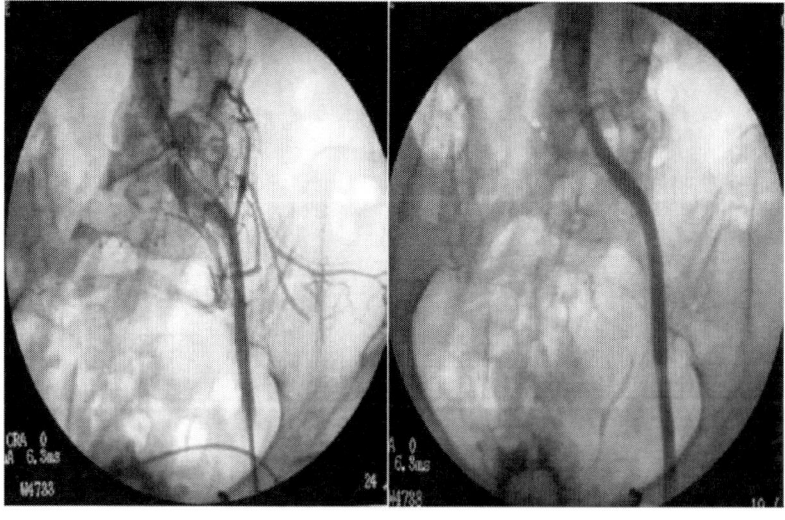

Figure 1. Case 1: 78y, Female, Left ilio-femoral venous thrombosis, the onset was 4 days ago. Wall stent was placed at the obstruction of left common iliac vein (iliac compression) after surgical thrombectomy. Left ilio-femoral venous region became clear after stenting.

Table 1. Ideas of preventing re-thrombosis after surgical thrombectomy

Establishment of temporary AV fistula
Clearance of ilio-femoral venous outflow using angioplasty and stenting
Adequate anticoagulation and compression therapy
Additional regional thrombolysis

Clinical Results

1. Complications of Surgical Thrombectomy

Pulmonary embolism is one of serious complications, but recent reports showed that fatal and symptomatic pulmonary embolism peri- and post-operative period is quite rare (less than 1%). [8-13, 16] A prospective randomized study showed the rate of additional pulmonary embolism detected using a perfusion scan after 1-4 weeks showed nosignificant difference between surgical thrombectomy and a conservatively treated group. [17]

Other reported uncommon complications were bleeding with hematoma, lymph leakage and infection in the groin [8-13].

2. Patency and Competency of Deep Vein after Thrombectomy

Re-thrombosis is the one of most important factors directly influencing surgical results through the long-term period and mostly occurs in early post-operative days [9, 11, 12]. According to collected data from 1984 to 1997 with 11 studies by Rutherford, Mewissen and Eklof, the patency rate of the iliac vein were 54% to 93%, average 77.3% [18]. The primary patency rate of recent reports with additional iliac endovascular therapy is from 74% to 81%. Secondary patency rate of iliac vein in long-term follow up is 84-91% (mean follow up periods, 22-68 months) [9-13]. The patency rate of the iliac vein after thrombectomy is as good as that after catheter-directed thrombolysis. [6]

Regarding femoro-popliteal venous lesions, the occlusion rate of the femoro-popliteal vein after operation is 10-39%, [11, 14], and the competency rate of the femoro-popliteal vein is 50-60% after 10 years, although the competency of the femoro-popliteal vein deteriorates over time after the operation [4, 16]. Also, it is reported that patent ilio-caval segments lead to better infra-inguinal patency, valvular competence and clinical symptoms [11].

In addition to clearance of ilio-femoral vein thrombus, complete removal of distal thrombus of the femoral vein may prevent re-thrombus of the iliac vein and keep competency of the femoro-popliteal vein.

3. Long Term Results of Venous Thrombectomy

A single 10-year follow-up study of comparison between surgical thrombectomy and conservative therapy showed that surgical thrombectomy had better clinical outcomes in early post-operative periods and in late post-operative periods compared to conservative therapy. Other long-term follow-up studies also showed good clinical outcomes [12, 16].

The Future of Surgical Thrombectomy

The evidence level for surgical venous thrombectomy for selected patients is IIb from the reports of ACCP guide line 2008. [1]

Current venous thrombectomy combined with endovenous therapy is expected to clear deep vein thrombus immediately and obtain better results over a classical thrombectomy [9-13]. However, these are single center studies with a small number of subjects, so compiling more data is needed to confirm the evidence level.

References

[1]   Kearon. C., Kahn, S.R., Agnelli, G., Goldhaber, S., Raskob, G.E., Comerota, A.J., et al. Anti-thrombotic therapy for venous thromboembolic disease: American College of Chest Physicians Evidence-Based Clinical Practice Guidelines (8th Edition). *Chest.* 2008; 133 (6 Suppl): 454-545S.

[2]   Cho, J.S., Martelli, E., Mozes, G., Miller, V.M., Gloviczki, P. Effects of thrombolysis and venous thrombectomy on valvular competence, thrombogenicity, venous wall morphology, and function. *J. Vasc. Surg.* 1998; 28: 787-99.

[3]   Comerota, A.J., Paolini, D. Treatment of acute ilio-femoral deep venous thrombosis: a strategy of thrombus removal. *Eur. J. Vasc. Endovasc. Surg.* 2007; 33: 351-60.

[4]   Plate, G., Eklof, B., Norgren, L., Ohlin, P., Dahlstrom, J.A. Venous thrombectomy for ilio-femoral vein thrombosis 10-year results of a prospective randomized study. *Eur. J. Vasc. Endovasc. Surg.* 1997; 4: 367-74.

[5]   Sillesen, H., Just, S., Jorgensen, M., Baekgaard, N. Catheter-directed thrombolysis for treatment of ilio-femoral deep venous thrombosis is durable, preserves venous valve function and may prevent chronic venous insufficiency. *Eur. J. Vasc. Endovasc. Surg.* 2005; 30: 556-62.

[6]   Mewissen, M.W., Seabrook, G.R., Meissner, M.H., Cynamon, J., Labropoulos, N., Haughton, S.H. Catheter-directed thrombolysis for lower extremity deep venous thrombosis: report of a national multicenter registry. *Radiology.* 1999; 211: 39-49.

[7]   Comerota, A.J., Gale, S.S. Technique of contemporary ilio-femoral and infra-inguinal venous thrombectomy. *J. Vasc. Surg.* 2006; 43: 185-91.

[8]   Eklof, B., Kamida, C.B., Kistner, R.L., Masuda, E.M. Contemporary treatment of ilio-femoral deep vein thrombosis. In *Perspectives in vascular surgery*, Thieme Medical publishers, New York, 1999. pp1-27.

[9]   Mickley, V., Schwagierek, R., Rilinger, N., Gorich, J., Sunder-Plassmann, L. Left iliac venous thrombosis caused by venous spur: treatment with thrombectomy and stent implantation. *J. Vasc. Surg.* 1998; 28: 492-7.

[10]   Schwarzbach, M.H.M., Schumacher, H., Bockler, D., Furstenberger, S., Thomas, F., Seelos, R., et al. Surgical thrombectomy followed by intraoperative endovascular reconstruction for symptomatic ilio-femoral venous thrombosis. *Eur. J. Vasc. Endovasc. Surg.* 2005; 29: 58-66.

[11]   Hartung, O., Benmiloud, F., Barthelemy, P., Dubuc, M., Boufi, M., Alimi, Y.S. Late results of surgical venous thrombectomy with ilio-caval stenting. *J. Vasc. Sur.g* 2008; 47: 381-7.

[12]   Holper, P., Kotelis, D., Attigah, N., Hylik-Durr, A., Bocker, D. Long-term results after surgical thrombectomy and simultaneous stenting for symptomatic ilio-femoral venous thrombosis. *Eur. J. Vasc. Endovasc. Surg.* 2010; 39: 349-55.

[13]   Blättler, W., Heller, G., Largiadèr, J., Savolainen, H., Gloor, B., Schmidli, J., et al. Combined regional thrombolysis and surgical thrombectomy for the treatment of ilio-femoral vein thrombosis. *J. Vasc. Surg.* 2004; 40: 620-5.

[14] Plate, G., Einarsson, E., Ohlin, P., Jensen, R., Qvarfordt, P., Eklof, B. Thrombectomy with temporary arteriovenous fistula: The treatment of choice in acute ilio-femoral venous thrombosis. *J. Vasc. Surg.* 1984; 1: 867-876.

[15] Ogawa, T., Hoshino, S., Midorikawa, H., Sato, K. Intermittent pneumatic compression of the foot and calf improves the outcome of catheter-directed thrombolysis using low-dose urokinase in patients with acute proximal venous thrombosis of the leg *J. Vasc. Surg.* 2005; 42: 940-944.

[16] Juhan, M.C., Alimi, Y.S., Barthelemy, P..J, Fabre, D.F., Riviere, C.D. Late results of ilio-femoral venous thrombectomy. *J. Vasc. Surg.* 1997; 25: 417-22.

[17] Plate, G., Ohlin, P., Eklof, B. Pulmonary embolism in acute ilio-femoral venous thrombosis. *Br. J. Surg.* 1985; 72: 912-5.

[18] Rutherford, R., Eklof, B., Mewissen, M. Interventional treatments for ilio-femoral venous thrombosis. In *Vascular Surgery* 5th edition, WB Saunders, Philadelphia, 2000, pp1959-68.

In: Deep Vein Thrombosis
Editor: Takashi Yamaki

ISBN: 978-1-62257-519-0
© 2013 Nova Science Publishers, Inc.

The Survey of Deep Vein Thrombosis and Venous Thromboembolism Prevention: Japanese Vein Study XIII

Hirono Satokawa[1,], Takashi Yamaki[2], Hirohide Iwata[3], Masahiro Sakata[4], Norihide Sugano[5], Toshiya Nishibe[6], Makoto Mo[7] and Norikazu Yamada[8]*

[1]Department of Cardiovascular Surgery, Fukushima Medical University, School of Medicine, Fukushima, Japan
[2]Department of Plastic and Reconstructive Surgery, Tokyo Women's Medical University, Tokyo, Japan
[3]Department of Vascular Surgery, Aichi Medical College, Nagakute, Japan
[4]Sakata Clinic, Osaka, Japan
[5]Department of Surgery, Tokyo Metropolitan Health and Medical Treatment Corporation Ohkubo Hospital, Tokyo, Japan
[6]Department of Cardiovascular Surgery, Tokyo Medical University Hachioji Medical Center, Tokyo, Japan
[7]Department of Cardiovascular Surgery, Yokohama Minami Kyosai Hospital, Yokohama, Japan

* Correspondence to: Hirono Satokawa M.D. Department of Cardiovascular Surgery, Fukushima Medical University, 1 Hikariga-oka, Fukushima City, Fukushima Prefecture, 960-1295 Japan. Tel: +81-24-547-1111. Fax: + 81-24-548-3926. E-mail: satokawa@fmu.ac.jp.

[8]Department of Cardiology, Mie University Graduate School
of Medicine, Tsu, Japan
The Committee for Survey of the Japanese Society
of Phlebology, Japan

Abstract

Several years have passed since the guidelines of venous thromboembolism (VTE) treatment and VTE prevention were published. The treatment of deep vein thrombosis (DVT) is changing greatly. This study was performed to investigate the risk factors, diagnostic methods, distribution, and treatment of DVT and to investigate VTE prevention in Japan. A questionnaire survey was mailed to the members of the Japanese Society of Phlebology. The contents of the survey dealt with the treatment of new DVT cases in the year 2009 and the prevention of VTE. The results were examined and compared to the result of our former survey. 1162 patients were reported from 70 institutions. The sex ratio (men to women) was 1 to 2 and the age ranged from 15 to 102 (average 69). Surgery was the most important risk factor for DVT (38.2%). As for the onset time, the acute onset (within 13 days) occurred in 486 patients (41.8%) and the subacute (14-29 days) in 70 (6.0%). Subsequent pulmonary thromboembolism was diagnosed in 174 patients (15.0%). For diagnosis, an ultrasound method was mainly used (87.7%), whereas phlebography was used for only 33 patients (2.8%). DVT was found in left lower limb in 531 patients (48.6%), in right lower limb in 360 patients (33.0%) and in bilateral limbs in 201 patients (18.4%). DVT locations were proximal type (52.2%) and distal type (47.8%), which included 119 patients with bilateral distal type. In the distal type, soleal vein thrombosis was most frequent (84.3%) and then peroneal vein thrombosis (19.9%). Patients were mainly treated medicinally (80.8%). Medication included unfractionated heparin (57.0%) and Urokinase (11.1%). Catheter-directed thrombectomy was performed in 22 cases (2.4%) and surgical thrombectomy was done only in 14 (1.6%). Vena cava filter was inserted for 155 patients (17.2%): retrievable type (66.5%), permanent type (21.3%) and temporary type (9.7%). Prophylactic methods were used at 60 institutions (85.7%). The precautions were elastic stockings (91.4%), early ambulation (84.3%), pneumatic compression (81.4%) and anticoagulant drugs (52.9%).

The number of DVT patients has increased and the frequency of the distal type especially increased. Anticoagulant therapy is most common medical treatment. The total frequency of vena cava filter was similar to our previous survey; however, the use ratio of retrievable type increased comparatively. Prophylactic methods for VTE were used in most institutions, however, the rate of anticoagulation administration was not high and is considered to be insufficient in Japan.

Introduction

Several years have already passed since the presentation of the guidelines for the diagnosis and treatment of pulmonary thromboembolism (PTE) and deep vein thrombosis (DVT) and for the prevention of venous thromboembolism (VTE) in Japan. [1, 2] During this time their incidence, treatment and prophylaxis have considerably changed. Some epidemiological surveys of DVT were performed in times past. In Japan, the Committee for the Survey of the Japanese Society of Phlebology performed a survey investigation of DVT in 1999 and in 2004. [3, 4] We have performed a cross-sectional multi-center survey of DVT 7 years after the second survey, analyzed the data and report the results.

Materials and Methods

A questionnaire survey was mailed to the about 800 active members of the Japanese Society of Phlebology. The questionnaire dealt with the treatment of new DVT cases in the year 2009 and the prevention of VTE. The contents of the questionnaire were about the diagnosis, risk factors, concomitant and subsequent diseases, distribution of VTE, the treatment (procedures, drugs) and the prophylaxis (performance rate, prophylactic procedures). The results were examined and compared to the result of the former surveys.

Results

Patients Number and Background

Seventy institutions responded and 1162 cases were reported. The sex ratio (men to women, which were recorded) was 383 to 761 and the age ranged from 15 to 102 (average 69). There was a peak of incidence in 80 year olds, and more frequent in 70 and then in 90 year olds. The number of DVT cases was from 1 to 267 (mean 17.9) per institute. According to onset time, 486 patients (41.8%) were acute type (within 13 days); 70 (6.0%) were subacute (14 to 29 days); 104 (9.0%) chronic type (over than 30 days); 464 (39.9%) unknown; and for 38 patients (3.3%) there was no record.

Characteristics of DVT Patients

Risk Factors (Table 1)

Answers to risk factors were multiple-choice. Surgery was selected in 444 patients (38.2%). Among types of surgery, 354 were orthopedic surgery (79.7%) (Total knee replacement 213, total hip replacement 43, others 98), digestive tract 23 (5.2%), vascular 13 (2.9%), gynecologic 11 (2.4%), urologic 9 (2.0%), cerebral 8 (1.8%), cardiac 5 (1.1%) and other surgery 21 (4.7%). Other risk factors were malignant disorder 192 (16.5%), immobilization 145 (12.5%), trauma 40 (3.4%), iliac compression 34 (2.9%), intravenous catheter 29 (2.5%), dehydration 27 (2.3%), cast fixation (1.3%), pregnancy 13 (1.1%) and long-flight 10 (0.9%).

In comparison with the 2nd survey, the rate of risk from surgery changed from 24% to 38%, a large difference. Concerning economy class (long-flight) syndrome, flight time was from 2 to 12 hours (mean 7.0) and there were 5 DVT patients immobilized by other long trips. In 617 patients (68.1%) there was only one risk factor. In 150 patients (16.6%) there were plural factors. Among patients with malignant disorder, 17 (8.9%) had colon cancer, uterus cancer 14 (7.3%), ovarian cancer 10 (5.2%), pulmonary cancer 8 (4.2%), prostate cancer 6 (3.1%), leukemia (including malignant lymphoma) 5 (2.6%) and others.

Concomitant and Subsequent Diseases

Patients complicated with PTE were 174 (15.0%) and that number was less than the 23% in the survey of 2004. Stroke coexisted in 43 patients (3.7%), chronic renal insufficiency in 8 (0.7%), atrial fibrillation in 8 (0.7%), thrombophlebitis of superficial vein in 5 (0.4%), systemic lupus erythematosus in 2 (0.2%). Inflammatory enteric disease was not present.

Table1. Specific risk factors for deep vein thrombosis

Risk factors	Patients No. (%) n=1162
Surgery	444 (38.2)
Malignant disorder	192 (16.5)
Immobilization	145 (12.5)
Trauma	40 (3.4)
Iliac compression	34 (2.9)
Intravenous catheter	29 (2.5)
Dehydration	27 (2.3)
Cast fixation	15 (1.3)
Pregnancy	13 (1.1)
Long flight	10 (0.9)

Incidence of Thrombophilia

This section of the survey was also multiple-choice. Protein S deficiency was most frequent, 23 patients (2.0%). Protein C deficiency, 12 patients (1.0%); positive lupus anticoagulant, 8 patients (0.7%); positive cardiolipin antibody, 8 patients (0.7%); and antithrombin III deficiency, 4 patients (0.3%). There were no patients with plasminogen abnormality or positive factor V Leiden. Incidences of thrombophilia were infrequent compared with the 2004' survey. We did not confirm whether examination of thrombophilia was performed in all patients and therefore the results might be affected. There were 22 patients complicated with connective tissue disease among whom 6 were taking steroids. Other special conditions were 74 patients (6.4%) with diabetes mellitus, 23 (2.0%) undergoing hormone replacement therapy and 13 (1.1%) undergoing steroid therapy.

Diagnosis of DVT

Procedure of Diagnosis (Figure 1)

Another multiple choice question. Ultrasound was used most frequently, in 1,020 patients (87.7%). Contrast CT was used in 457 (39.3%), phlebography in 33 (2.8%), plethysmography 25 (2.1%) and MRI 16 (1.4%). Compared to our 2004 survey, the use of ultrasound changed from 70%.

Contrast CT slightly increased, and phlebography decreased from 38% to 2.8%, remarkably. Concerning a combination of diagnostic procedures, a pair of procedures was performed for 394 patients (33.9%), in among which ultrasound plus contrast CT was most often used, 354 patients (30.5%). For 20 patients (1.7%) three procedures for diagnosis were performed.

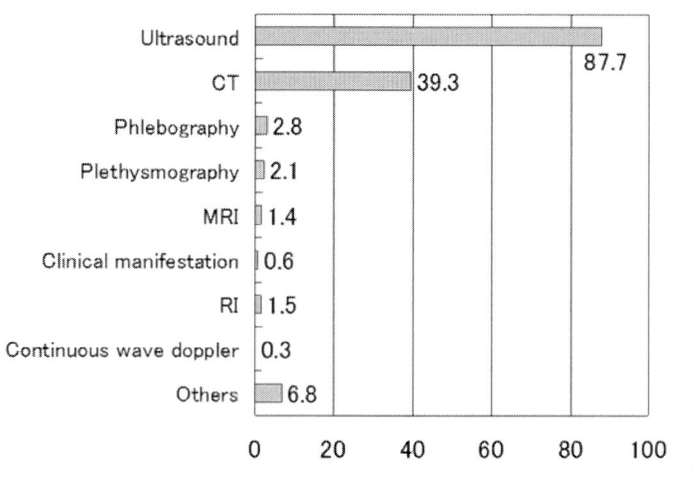

Figure 1. Diagnostic methods for deep vein thrombosis.

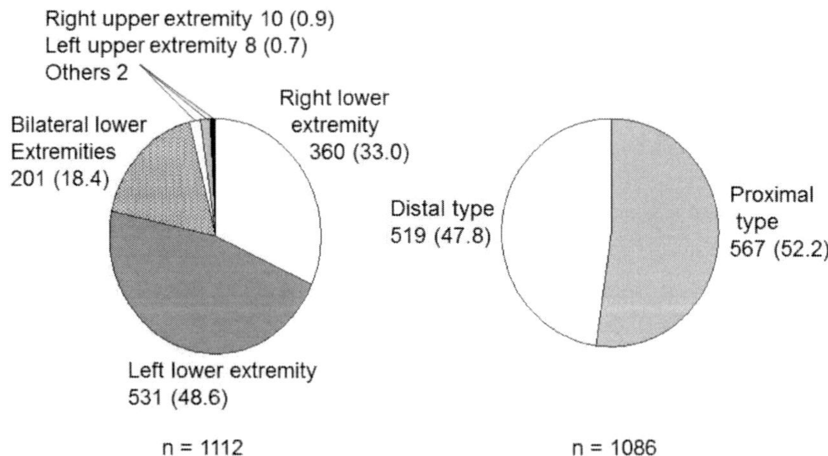

Figure 2. Distribution of deep vein thrombosis.

Distribution of DVT (Figure 2)

Distribution of DVT was recorded for 1112 patients. There were 1092 patients with lower extremity DVT among whom 360 with DVT in right lower extremity (33.0%), in left lower extremity 531 (48.6%) and in bilateral lower extremities 201 (18.4%). Incidence of bilateral lower extremities DVT increased compared to the 2004 survey. Anatomic distribution of 1086 patients was recorded in this study. DVT distribution was classified as proximal type where the thrombus was present at the central part from the popliteal vein and distal type where DVT ranged in the calf vein. Proximal type were 567 patients (52.2%), distal type were 519 (47.8%). The patients whose thrombus was present from the distal side to the proximal side vein accounted for 188 patients, which was 33.2% of proximal type DVT. Among the proximal type, DVT from the calf vein to the popliteal vein occurred in 84 patients (14.8%), and there were 52 patients with DVT in the popliteal vein (9.2%), 41 with DVT in the femoral vein (7.2%). Total limbs of distal type DVT were 638 among which there were 119 bilateral patients. The thrombus was found in the soleal vein in 538 patients (84.3%); in the peroneal vein in 127 (19.9%); in the posterior tibial vein in 78 (12.2%); in the gastrocnemial vein in 49 patients (7.7%) and in the anterior tibial vein in 3 patients (0.5%). (Figure 3)

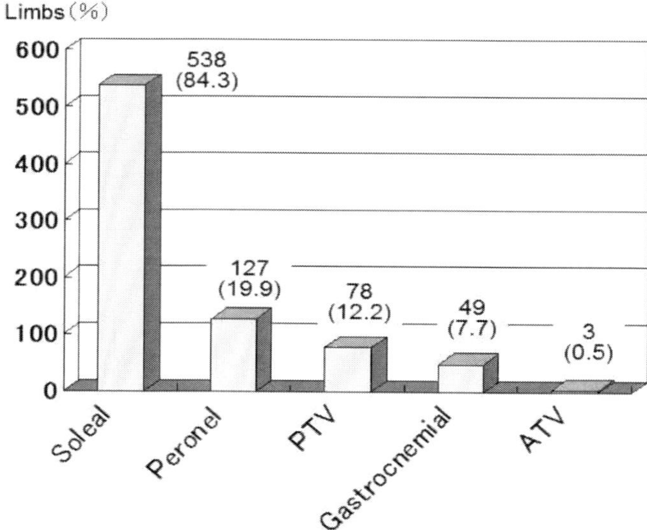

PTV: posterior tibial vein, ATV: anterior tibial vein.

Figure 3. Distribution of distal type deep vein thrombosis.

Table 2. Medicinal treatment for deep vein thrombosis

Total cases		Patients No. (%) n=901
Medicinal treatment		728 (80.8)
Unfractionated heparin		514 (57.0)
Dose	3,000-38,400 (mean 13,137) U/day	
Duration	1-50 (mean 8.9) day	
Low molecular weight heparin		36 (4.0)
Urokinase		100 (11.1)
Dose	12,000-960,000 (mean 366,093) U/day	
Duration	1-16 (mean 5.7) day	
Tissue plasminogen activator		15 (1.7)
Warfarin		981 (75.6)
PT-INR	1.0-3.1 (mean 1.9)	

Treatment

Every treatment was recorded and we received the record of treatment given to 901 patients.

Medicinal Treatment (Table 2)

Medicinal treatment was given to 728 patients (80.8%). The anticoagulant agent, unfractionated heparin (UFH) was injected to 514 patients (57.0%) and low molecular weight heparin (LMWH) to 36 patients (4.0%). 3,000 to 38,400/units/day (mean 13,137) of UFH was administered, with duration of from 1 to 50 days (mean 8.9). LMWH was most often used with enoxaparin sodium. In addition, 21 patients (2.3%) were injected with fondaparinux and 6 patients (0.7%) with argatroban. As for oral anticoagulant drugs, warfarin was given to 981 patients (75.6%), which were monitored by international normalized ratio of prothrombin time (PTINR) (1.0 − 3.1 (mean 1.9)) at 61 institutes and by thrombotest (3 − 84 % (mean 35)) at 49 institutes. Average duration of warfarin administration was 5.8 months. Patients taking aspirin were only 23 (2.6%). Concerning thrombolytic agents, urokinase was used for 100 patients (11.1%) and monteplase was administered to only 15 patients (1.7%). Dosage of urokinase ranged from 12,000 to 960,000 U/day (mean 366,093) and administered from 1 to 16 days (mean 5.7).

Table 3. Surgical treatment for deep vein thrombosis

	Patients No. (%)
Total cases	n=901
Surgical treatment	14 (1.6)
Thrombectomy	14 (1.6)
Thrombectomy plus stent	7 (0.8)
Bypass operation	2 (0.2)
A-V shunt	1 (0.1)
Ligation of vein	0 (0)

Table 4. Endovascular treatment for deep vein thrombosis

	Patients No. (%)
Total cases	n=901
Endovascular treatment	162 (18.0)
Catheter-directed thrombosis	22 (2.4)
Stent	3 (0.3)
IVC filter	155 (17.2)
Retrievable type	103 (66.5)
Permanent type	33 (21.3)
Temporary type	15 (9.7)
No record	4 (2.6)

Table 5. Conservative treatment for deep vein thrombosis

	Patients No. (%)
Total cases	n=901
Conservative treatment	879 (97.6)
Elastic stocking	799 (88.7)
Elastic bandage	152 (16.9)
Elevation of lower limbs	185 (20.5)
Bed rest	79 (8.8)

Surgical Treatment (Table 3)

We classified VCF insertion as endovascular surgery. Thrombectomy was performed in only 14 patients (1.6%). Among of these 14, a stent was inserted in 7 patients (0.8%) . Bypass surgery was performed for 2 patients (0.2%), and construction of an A-V fistula was done for 1 (0.1%). There was no patient with vein ligation.

Endovascular Treatment (Table 4)

Inferior vena cava filter (VCF) was inserted for 155 patients (17.2%). Patients with VCF consisted of 103 patients with retrievable type (66.5%), 33 patients with permanent type (21.3%) and 15 patients with temporary type (9.7%). Modalities of VCF were as follows: 71 patients received Günther tulip[TM] (Cook Medical, Bloomington, USA); 26, OptEase[TM] (Cordis, Tokyo, Japan); 15, TrapEase[TM] (Cordis, Tokyo, Japan); 9 , NeuhausProtect[TM] (Toray Medical, Tokyo, Japan); 4, LGM30D/U[TM] (B.Braun Medical, Boulogne, France) and others. Endovascular surgery, besides the above-mentioned, thrombectomy or stent deployment was performed for 25 patients (2.7%). This consisted of catheter-directed thrombolysis (CDT) in 22 patients (2.4%) and stent deployment in 3 patients (0.3%). Among of endovascular treatments, there were patients who were treated by CDT plus VCF in 17 patients (1.9%) and by CDT plus stent in 1 patient (0.1%).

Table 6. Onset, anatomical distribution and treatments

Onset	Acute-subacute group		Chronic group	
Distribution	Proximal DVT N=388	Distal DVT N=145	Proximal DVT N=196	Distal DVT N=387
Medicinal treatment	359 (92.5)	118 (81.3)	141 (71.9)	89 (23.0)
UFH	286 (73.7)	73 (50.3)	95 (48.5)	36 (9.3)
Warfarin	330 (85.1)	108 (74.5)	139 (70.9)	75 (19.4)
Surgical treatment	14 (3.6)	0 (0)	0 (0)	0 (0)
Endovascular treatment	130 (33.5)	8 (5.5)	24 (12.2)	0 (0)
IVC filter	116 (29.9)	8 (5.5)	22 (11.2)	3 (0.8)
CDT	18 (4.6)	0 (0)	3 (1.5)	0 (0)
Stent	0 (0)	0 (0)	2 (1.0)	0 (0)
Conservative treatment	311 (80.3)	92 (63.4)	152 (77.6)	295 (76.2)
ES	274 (70.6)	83 (57.2)	138 (70.4)	284 (73.4)

UFH: unfractionated heparin, IVC: inferior vena cava, CDT: catheter-directed thrombolysis, ES: elastic stockings.

Conservative Treatment (Table 5)

This section of the questionnaire was also multiple-choice. Conservative treatment was selected for 879 patients (97.6%). Procedures were elastic stockings as compression treatment for 799 patients (88.7%), elastic bandage for 152 patients (16.9%), elevation of lower limbs for 185 patients (20.5%) and bed rest for 79 patients (8.8%).

DVT Onset and Treatments (Table 6)

Patients, who had distinct record of the onset type and of the distribution, were divided according to the onset period: acute-subacute group, onset within 29 days; chronic group, onset more than 30 days and unknown group. There were 533 patients in the acute-subacute group; proximal type 388 and distal type 145, and 583 patients in the chronic group; proximal type 196 and distal type 387. For the proximal type DVT of the acute-subacute group medicinal treatment was selected for 92.5% of the patients and warfarin was administered to 85.1% of these. On the other hand, medicinal treatment was selected for 23.0% and warfarin administration rate was only 19.4% for the distal type of the chronic group. Surgical treatment was done mainly on proximal type of acute-subacute group. VCF was mainly chosen for proximal type of the acute-subacute group; however it was deployed in 22 patients (11.2%) with proximal type of the chronic group. Other endovascular treatment was selected for 4.6% patients of proximal type of the acute-subacute group and for 2.5% of proximal type of the chronic group.

Prophylaxis of DVT

Answers were received from 70 institutes. The Japanese guidelines for prevention of VTE [1] were well known to 66 institute doctors (94.3%). Sixty-three institutes answered that unified prophylactic methods were necessary to prevent VTE. There were 60 institutes that actually used prophylactic methods. Of these, treatment was unified at the whole institute in 29 (41.4%) and dependent on each department in 30 institutions (42.8%). After the induction of prophylaxis 29 institutions (41.4%) answered that VTE decreased, 16 institutions reported no change and 4 saw VTE increase. Prophylactic methods were elastic stockings at 64 institutions (91.4%), pneumatic compression at 57 (81.4%), early ambulation at 59 (84.3%), self-exercise at 44 (62.9%) and anticoagulant agents administered at 37 (52.9%). As for anticoagulant drugs, UFH was administered at 26 institutions (37.1%), LMWH at 16 (22.9%) and fondaparinux at 16 (22.9%). Institutions, that evaluate patient's VTE risk and use proper prophylactic methods for high-risk and low-risk patients, were 53 (75.7%). Other 11 institutions (15.7%)

performed prophylaxis without distinguishing patient's risk. 40 institutions (57.1%) administered UFH to high or highest risk patients following Japanese guidelines.

Discussion

The incidence of DVT increased to 17.9 patients per institution compared to 10 patients in 1999 and 9.9 in 2004. [3,4]. The other survey in Japan by Japanese Society of Pulmonary Embolism Research (JASPER) revealed that estimated DVT patients were 14,674 annually in 2004 (12 patients / 100,000 persons). [5, 6] In this study, the average age of DVT patients was 69.1; however, the peak was at 80 years, older than the peak age in the 2004 survey. Concerning the onset phase of DVT, the rate of acute-subacute decreased to about 48% from 62% in the 1999 survey. On the other hand patients in the chronic group including those of unknown of onset increased to 43.2% from 34% in 1999.

Surgery as a risk factor was 38.2% compared to 16 % in the 1999 survey and 23.9% in 2004. Other risk factors did not change greatly. We know that DVT occurs at high rate on occasion of surgery and it was reported that DVT occurred in about 25% of the patients in general surgery and more frequently in orthopedics surgery. [7] On the contrary according to the study done by JASPER, PTE resulting from major surgery gradually decreased. [5] Concomitance of PTE from DVT was 15%, a decrease from the our former survey. I thought that the increase of chronic phase and the increase of distal type DVT might affect the incidence of PTE.

For diagnosis of DVT, ultrasound use increased to 87.7% in this study from 23% in 1999 and from 70% in 2004. Contrast CT was at 39.3%. To diagnose DVT, imaging examinations were necessary and verification of thrombus is important. Ultrasound has the advantage of being simple, easy, repeatable and has a high diagnosis precision. [8] Therefore ultrasound is recommended as the 1st choice for DVT diagnosis. [7] CT needs contrast media for DVT diagnosis; however it has developed as superior in fine spatial resolution which can examine not only full length limb but also pulmonary artery in a short time and is popularly available. [9, 10] On the other hand, phlebography which was once considered to be the gold standard examination for DVT, is invasive and its use has become less frequent, only 2.8% in this survey. In the diagnosis of acute DVT the indication for phlebography is now selective: when the ultrasound is not definitive, where iliofemoral venous thrombosis exists and thrombectomy is planned and when catheter-directed thrombolysis is being considered. [11]

Concerning DVT distribution, distal type increased from 16% in 2004 to 47.8% in this survey. Incidences of distal DVT were reported at 15%-47% and emphasized the recent increase. [12, 13] In distal DVT, soleal vein thrombosis occurred in 84% of the patients. This result coincided with reports that indicated that calf thrombus occurred most frequently in the soleal vein. [14, 15]

Medicinal treatment for DVT was mainly anticoagulation drugs, among which UFH administration decreased to 57.0% compared to 61.2% in the 2004 survey and warfarin was administered at the same level. Intake of warfarin was controlled by PT-INR in 67% of the institutions and average controlled PT-INR was 1.9, which was same as our former survey. PT-INR count was lower than the 2.0-3.0 recommended by ACCP evidence-based clinical practice guidelines [16] and was equivalent to the Japanese guidelines. [2] Use frequency of LMWH was about the same, and fondaparinux, a new anticoagulation drug, was used for 2.3% of the patients. Urokinase administration decreased to 11.1% from 49% in the 2004 survey. It was reported that thrombolytic treatment reduced DVT recurrence and postthrombotic syndrome. However, we assume that the recommendation level of Class IIb might affect the choice of treatment. [2, 16]

Surgical treatment such as thrombectomy or bypass surgery became less frequent compared with the 2004 survey and endovascular treatment excluding VCF decreased to CDT in 2.4% and stent deployment in 0.3%. Increase of chronic or of distal DVT might be the reason for the decrease of surgical and endovascular treatments. VCF deployment was the most common endovascular treatment for DVT. The ratio of the treatment did not greatly change from 2004. The retrievable type accounted for 66.5% of the VCF's and the use of the permanent type decreased. It was reported that DVT recurrence increased 2 years after VCF insertion [17] which suggests that the retrievable type VCF should be removed as much as possible. However the retrieval rate of retrievable type VCF is not always 100%. [18] On the other hand, temporary VCF has problems such as fixation of catheter shaft, risk of infection and necessity of counterplan when major thrombus trapping occurs. [19]

Conservative treatment was used in 97.6% of the patients, a large increased from the 69.8% of the 2004 survey. Among conservative treatments, elastic stockings were used for 88.7% of the patients. It is controversial whether the compression by elastic stockings increases PE risk or whether early ambulation with elastic stockings can improve the symptoms. [2] The DVT treatments were different according to the DVT onset phases. Severe static proximal DVT in acute onset will need aggressive treatment such as surgery or catheter intervention. Chronic DVT was treated with mainly conservative treatments including compression therapy. This strategy for DVT treatment was supported by our study results. Especially it became clear that compression therapy by elastic stockings is the main conservative treatment.

The Japanese Guidelines for Prevention of VTE were published and the 2nd edition has already been reported [2] according to the ACCP. There were several reports that DVT decreased when prophylactic procedures including anticoagulant drugs were developed. [21, 22] However, the rate of following these guidelines is relatively low. [22] According to our survey the guidelines were known by 94.3% of the respondents, but only 85.7% of the institutions performed prophylactic procedures. Since April 2004, DVT prophylaxis as prevention of VTE has been covered by national medical insurance in Japan. This has given incentive to prophylaxis use. But further effort is necessary to educate doctors in the guidelines and the importance of prophylaxis. Elastic stockings were the most common prophylaxis procedure. However, anticoagulant treatment including UFH, which is recommended for high risk patients, was administered to only 52.9% of the patients. Anticoagulant drugs besides UFH are not recommended for prophylaxis by the Japanese guidelines. Fondaparinux was quiet recently permitted to both DVT treatment and VTE prophylaxis, and LMWH are permitted as prophylaxis use only after orthopedic or abdominal surgery by Japanese medical insurance. In this survey about 20% institutions used these drugs.

In conclusion, our study provides characteristics and the prophylaxis of the DVT in Japan. DVT cases increased, especially distal type. Medicinal treatment was mainly anticoagulant therapy. Retrievable type VCFs were most often inserted. DVT prophylaxis is not known to all medical personnel. The rate of anticoagulation therapy is not high. Therefore further study and effort is needed to instruct doctors about the use of prophylaxis.

Acknowledgment

We express our gratitude to the participant institutions and to the doctors. This paper is to be published in the Japanese Journal of Phlebology.

References

[1]   Editorial Committee on Japanese Guideline for Prevention of Venous Thromboembolism. Japanese Guideline for Prevention of Venous Thromboembolism. Medical Front International Limited, Tokyo (2004).

[2]   JCS Joint Working Group. Guidelines for the Diagnosis, Treatment and Prevention of Pulmonary Thromboembolism and Deep Vein Thrombosis (JCS2009). *Circ. J.* 75, 1258-81 (2011).

[3]   Hoshino S, Satokawa H. Deep vein thrombosis; Japanese Vein Study I. *Jpn. J. Phlebol.* 8, 307-11 (1997).

[4]   Yamaki T, Hirai M, Oota T, et al. Deep vein thrombosis; Japanese Vein Study VII. *Jpn. J. Phlebol.* 15, 79-84 (2004).

[5]   Nakamura M, Sakuma M, Yamada N, et al: Risk factors of acute pulmonary thromboembolism in Japanese patients hospitalized for medical illness: results of a multicenter registry in the Japanese society of pulmonary embolism research. *J. Thromb. Thrombolysis.* 21, 131-5 (2006).

[6]   Sakuma M, Nakamura M, Yamada N, et al. Venous thromboembolism-deep vein thrombosis with pulmonary embolism, deep vein thrombosis alone, pulmonary embolism alone. *Circ. J.* 73, 305-9 (2009).

[7]   Nicolaides AN, Fareed J, Kakkar AK, et al. Prevention and treatment of venous thromboembolism International Consensus Statement (Guideline according to scientific evidence). *Int. Angiol.* 25, 101-61 (2006).

[8]   Comerota AJ, Katz ML, Greenwald LL, et al. Venous duplex imaging: should it replace hemodynamic tests for deep venous thrombosis? *J. Vasc. Surg.* 11, 53-61 (1990).

[9]   Perrier A, Roy PM, Sanchez O, et al: Multidetector-row/computed tomography in suspected pulmonary embolism. *N. Engl. J. Med.* 352, 1760-68 (2005).

[10]   Salvolini L, Scaglione M, Giuseppetti GM, et al. Suspected pulmonary embolism and deep venous thrombosis: a comprehensive MDCT diagnosis in the acute clinical setting. *Eur. J. Radiol.* 65, 340-9 (2008).

[11]   Kamida CB, Kistner RL, Eklof B, et al. Lower extremity ascending and descending phlebography. In *Hand book of venous disorders*, 2nd edition, Gloviczki P, Yao JST eds, Arnold, 2001 (London, United Kingdom) pp.133-9.

[12] Seintureier C, Bosson JL, Colonna M, et al. Site and clinical outcome of deep vein thrombosis of the lower limbs: an epidemiological study. *J. Thromb. Haemost.* 3, 1362-7 (2005).

[13] Kearon C, Julian JA, Newman TE, et al. Noninvasive diagnosis of deep vein thrombosis. *Ann. Intern. Med.* 128, 663-7 (1998).

[14] Browse NL, Burnand KG, Irvine AT, et al. Deep vein thrombosis: pathology and diagnosis. Browse NL, et al.eds, *Diseases of the Veins*, Arnold, 1999 (London, United Kingdom), pp.249-91.

[15] Ohgi S, Tachibana M, Ikebuchi M, et al. Pulmonary embolism in patients with isolated soleal vein thrombosis. *Angiology.* 49, 759-64 (1998).

[16] Kearon C, Kahn SR, Agnelli G, et al. Antithrombotic therapy for venous thrombotic disease: American college of chest physicians evidence-based clinical practice guidelines (8th edition). *Chest.* 133, 454s-545s (2008).

[17] Decousus H, Leizorovicz A, Parent F, et al. A clinical trial of vena caval filters in the prevention of pulmonary embolism in patients with proximal deep-vein thrombosis: Prevention du Risque d'Embolie Pulmpnaire par Interruption Cave Study Group. *N. Engl. J. Med.* 338, 409-415 (1998).

[18] Berczi V, Bottomley JR, Thomas SM, et al. Long-term retrievability of IVC filters: should we abandon permanent devices? *Cardiovasc. Intervent. Radiol.* 30, 820-7 (2007).

[19] Task force on Pulmonary Embolism, European Society of Cardiology. Guidelines on diagnosis and management of acute pulmonary embolism. *Eur. Heart. J.* 21, 1301-36 (2000).

[20] Niimi K, Kobayashi M, Narita H, Yamamoto K, Komori K. Evaluation of the efficacy of venous thromboembolism prophylaxis guideline implementation in Japan. *Surgery. Today.* 40, 1129-1136 (2010).

[21] Nutescu EA. Assessing, preventing, and treating venous thromboembolism: evidence-based approaches. *Am. J. Health. Syst. Pharm.* 64 (11 Suppl 7), S5-13 (2007).

[22] Abdel-Razeq H, Albadainah F, Hijjawi S, et al. Venous thromboembolism (VTE) in hospitalized cancer patients: prophylaxis failure or failure to prophylax! *J. Thromb. Thrombolysis.* 31, 107-112 (2011).

Contributing Authors

Jennifer Foglietta MD
Medical Oncology Department, S.Maria della Misericordia Hospital,
Perugia, Italy

Mario Ganau MD, MSBM
Department of Neurosurgery, University Hospital Trieste, Trieste, Italy

Mehmet Kurtoglu MD
Department of General Surgery, Istanbul University, Istanbul School
of Medicine, Capa-Istanbul, Turkey

C. Rinaldi A. Lesmana MD
Department of Internal Medicine, Cipto Mangunkusumo Hospital
Medical Faculty, University of Indonesia, Jakarta, Indonesia

Tomohiro Ogawa MD
Department of Cardiovascular Surgery,
Fukushima Daiichi Hospital, Fukushima, Japan

Pinjala Ramakrishna MS, FRCSEd, FICS
Department of Vascular Surgery, Nizam's Institute of Medical Sciences,
Hyderabad, AP, India

Hirono Satokawa MD
Department of Cardiovascular Surgery, Fukushima Medical University,
School of Medicine, Fukushima, Japan

Takashi Yamaki MD
Department of Plastic and Reconstructive Surgery, Tokyo Women's Medical
University, Tokyo, Japan

Index

F

false negative, 63
false positive, 63
FDA, 25
fetus, 46
fiber, 78
fibrin, viii, 2, 4, 16, 60, 61, 67, 106
fibrinogen, 12, 37, 39, 45
fibrinolysis, 17, 30
fibrinolytic, vii, 1, 61
filters, 28, 44, 52, 56, 73, 74, 75, 105, 117, 142
fixation, 130, 131, 139
flight, 130, 131
force, 84, 142
formation, 19, 37, 73, 85, 107
fractures, 47, 56
fragments, 16
France, 136
fresh frozen plasma, xiii, 95, 111, 118

G

gangrene, 73, 120
general anesthesia, xiv, 37, 120, 121
general surgery, 41, 92, 97, 138
genes, xiii, 94
genetic factors, vii, 1
genetic predisposition, 106
Germany, 61
glioma, 27, 32, 47, 50, 53, 54
glutamate, 97
Gori, v, 11
growth factor, 18, 19
guidelines, xiv, 29, 43, 49, 56, 80, 101, 128, 129, 137, 139, 140, 142

H

half-life, viii, 2, 22, 74, 98, 107, 114
head injury, 43
head trauma, 28, 42, 54

heart failure, xii, 94
hematoma, 15, 47, 48, 123
hemiparesis, 38
hemiplegia, 38
hemophilia, 113
hemorrhage, xiii, 51, 53, 55, 94, 106, 111, 112, 118
hemostasis, 48, 113
heparin, viii, ix, xii, xv, 2, 7, 21, 23, 27, 32, 33, 35, 38, 40, 41, 44, 48, 49, 50, 51, 52, 53, 54, 55, 72, 74, 76, 85, 87, 88, 89, 90, 91, 92, 94, 95, 97, 99, 107, 114, 115, 128, 134, 136
high risk patients, 140
hip replacement, 97, 115, 130
histidine, 21
history, ix, 12, 18, 39, 44, 65, 78, 82, 101, 106
homocysteine, 104
Hong Kong, 52
hormone, vii, 1, 20, 78, 102, 131
hospitalization, 12, 24, 46
human, 16, 68, 98, 114
hypersensitivity, 107
hypertension, vii, 1, 81
hypomagnesemia, 18

I

idiopathic, 8, 78, 103, 117
images, 16
immobilization, ix, 6, 12, 13, 36, 45, 59, 78, 89, 102, 130
immunoglobulin, 23
improvements, 28, 80, 85, 115
in vitro, 102
incidence, vii, ix, x, 1, 2, 3, 5, 7, 8, 12, 17, 18, 25, 27, 35, 36, 37, 38, 41, 42, 43, 48, 51, 55, 58, 65, 73, 74, 78, 83, 84, 89, 90, 95, 104, 105, 111, 129, 138
India, 93, 97, 143
individuals, 73, 85, 101, 103, 117
Indonesia, 1, 143
induction, 99, 137
induction period, 99

Q

R

S